Go Faster Food

for runners, cyclists, swimmers and rowers

Kate Percy

Vermilion
LONDON

This edition first published in the UK in 2009 by Vermilion, an imprint of Ebury Publishing

Ebury Publishing is a Random House Group company

The Random House Group Limited Reg. No. 954009

Addresses for companies within the Random House Group can be found at www.randomhouse.co.uk

A CIP catalogue record for this book is available from the British Library

Penguin Random House is committed to a sustainable future for our business, our readers and our planet. This book is made from Forest Stewardship Council® certified paper.

Book designed and set by seagulls.net
Printed and bound in Great Britain by Clays Ltd, St Ives plc

ISBN 978 0 091 92932 9

Copies are available at special rates for bulk orders. Contact the sales development team on 020 7840 8487 for more information.

To buy books by your favourite authors and register for offers, visit www.randomhouse.co.uk

I would like to dedicate this book to my dear friend, Julie, in appreciation of the many hours she has spent cycling alongside me on my long endurance runs, keeping me company and providing me with flapjacks, drinks, laughter and gentle encouragement.

Acknowledgements

My thanks go to ...

- my husband Mark, who got me into running in the first place and whose steadfast support for *Go Faster Food* has never faltered
- my children Helena, James and William, for their patience and encouragement and, of course, for testing all the recipes
- Sue Baic, my brilliant and supportive nutritionist and the Department of Sport, Exercise and Health at Bristol University
- Nick Rose, our local Olympian, and David Castle of *Running Fitness*, for giving me such fantastic assistance in getting the book off the ground
- Laura Morris, my publishing agent, for her belief in the potential of *Go Faster Food*, and Kate Hordern, for pointing me in the right direction
- all my athlete friends and contacts, both elite and non-elite, for sharing their interesting eating and training habits
- my mum and dad, for their hawk-eyed proofreading and for kindling my interest in food and cooking in the first place

contents

foreword by liz yelling

Double Olympian; Commonwealth bronze medallist in the Marathon

As a double Olympian, being the best you can be is not just about training hard. It is also about all the little things that make a big difference. For me, healthy eating and making the right food choices has always been instrumental to better running performance. It is just as important as my training and inextricably linked to it. Great food helps me train, race and recover stronger and faster.

Go Faster Food provides active people, serious or recreational, with hands-on, practical advice about how to eat for good athletic performance. It describes why a healthy and nutritious diet is vital for optimal participation and better training, racing and competition. Its easy-to-understand approach makes it a must-read for those looking to improve their general diet, but also those looking to shave extra minutes off their best time. What makes this book great is that it's not just another book on why exercisers, athletes and people passionate about their health should make the right food choices; it also contains hundreds of great food recipes to put that theory into good real life practice. It's an essential piece for your running kitbag; a manual to eating well.

I love healthy eating and get great enjoyment from preparing a meal from fresh wholesome ingredients. Like most people I have a limited repertoire of recipes and I am very excited about adding to my diet with some new recipe ideas from *Go Faster Food.* The Turkish Turlu Turlu with couscous and tahini sauce and the American blueberry pancakes are two recipes I can't wait to try. I am also pleased to see two of my favourite treats included, just with better names: the 'go faster carrot cake' and the 'recovery rice pudding'.

Enjoy cooking up some better sporting performances with this great book!

introduction

'Man ist was man isst' – 'You are what you eat'. I would never have believed that these words would ring so true when I used them for my German thesis in those heady days as a student in southern Germany in the 80s. The nearest I came to sport then was a few leisurely descents of the local ski slope to the café for a glass of wine and a cheese fondue. How things have changed. I fell in love with a sports fanatic, married him and, despite several years of dragging my feet, ended up an enthusiastic and capable marathon runner.

This happened by accident really. Faced with the dreariness of watching my husband train for and run yet another marathon, I decided that enough was enough; I had to see for myself what all the fuss was about. After a few weeks of running two to three times a week, I started to really enjoy myself. I felt less stressed, more positive and full of energy. I decided to go the whole hog and to train for the New York Marathon.

Since then I haven't looked back. I have run the New York, Amsterdam, Berlin and London Marathons and now have a good enough qualifying time for entry into prestigious marathons like Boston. I also love running half marathons and cross-country races and I have even tried my hand at fell running. If I were a better swimmer I would be very tempted to have a go at triathlon, but I'll have to work on that one ...

I find that the main problem with doing all this exercise is fuelling the body adequately. Athletes, whether amateur or elite, really do have unique nutritional demands. When we are training, we can be burning up to several thousand calories every day. No wonder we get hungry. We can, and we should, eat more than the average person. Eating and drinking properly needs to become an essential part of our everyday routine and sticking to a good diet, especially in those hard-training weeks leading up to an event, can not only have a dramatic effect on stamina and performance, but it can also make our training easier and even help the body repair and improve itself.

I became interested in the best foods to eat for endurance a few years back, when my husband was training for New York in 2000. His training started well, but he gradually began to sound like a stuck record, complaining every day that he was tired and hungry and yawning constantly. I decided to study nutrition, I changed our diet and, like magic, he began to feel more energised and started to really enjoy his running.

I have become increasingly fascinated by how some foods help endurance and recovery better than others and why, when you lapse for just one day, you start to feel lethargic, your energy levels drop dramatically and you are unable to fulfil your potential. What is also so interesting is that it is not just ***what*** you eat and drink that is important, it is also ***how much*** you eat and ***when*** you eat it.

It is true that fuelling your body every day during training can get tedious, and career and family commitments often make following a healthy diet a real struggle. But you don't have to stick to the same old mountains of pasta and tins of tuna! As my own family has become more involved in sport – I also have three children who train most days – I have learned to create healthy, imaginative and delicious food combinations to help keep our energy levels topped up.

With *Go Faster Food* I would like to add a little zest to your training with my selection of tasty and original energy-boosting recipes. I hope to inspire you to think about what to eat and how much, when to eat it and why. Nutritious and delicious food should help you achieve your training goals with a smile on your face and a properly fuelled body so that you can push yourself that extra mile, faster. I hope you enjoy the recipes and I hope they make you feel good. Happy training!

Part One

nutrition and training

1

eat well, train well

What makes a healthy training diet? The answer – regular and varied meals that are high in carbohydrate, relatively low in fat and well balanced with protein, fibre, vitamins and minerals. There you have it; it's not rocket science. Listen to your body – if you are training hard and you feel hungry, you probably need to eat more. Try to cook as many meals as you can from scratch – it will save you money and you'll know exactly what's in them, avoid processed foods as much as possible, and take a relaxed attitude of 'everything in moderation', rather than getting too obsessed about calories or your exact intake of certain foods. This will help you to stay focussed, feel good, exercise better and enjoy your training without starting to feel that it is a chore.

The Go Faster route to healthy, happy training – five basic rules

1. Eat a balanced diet, eat when you are hungry and listen to your body

Training burns a vast amount of calories. Average weekly mileages vary according to your training schedule, but training for a triathlon or a marathon can easily burn between 3,000 and 5,000 extra calories a week, even more for some. It is important, therefore, to listen to your body and to eat when you are hungry. Try your best to fuel yourself with 'good', unprocessed calories. Your diet should be made up of around 60 per cent carbohydrate – that's bread, cereal, potatoes, pasta, rice, fruit and vegetables; 15 per cent from protein; and the rest from fat.

The Food Standards Agency (FSA) illustrates this very clearly with their Eatwell plate:

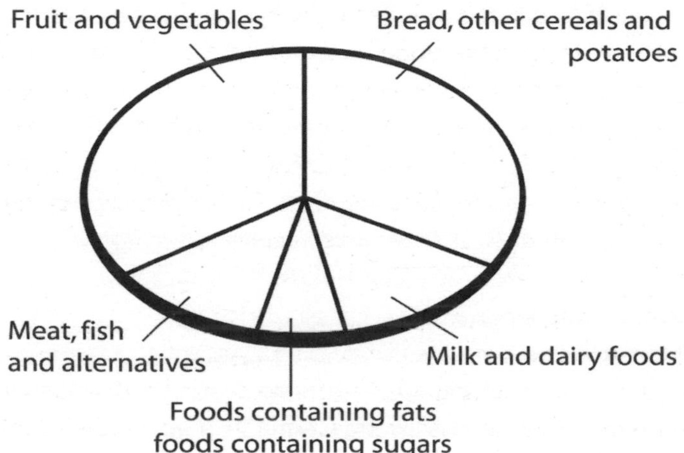

As an athlete, and especially if you are a female athlete, you also need to increase your intake of vitamins, iron and other minerals. Try to eat three meals a day and limit your snacks to healthy ones (pitta bread and hummus, oatcakes and peanut butter, nuts and seeds, fresh, canned or dried fruit, a few squares of dark chocolate, cereal bars or malt loaf).

2. Keep your hydration levels constant

Don't just drink before, during and after a training session. It is best to keep your hydration levels topped up all the time. If you wait until you feel thirsty, you will already be slightly dehydrated. Keep a bottle of water with you (tap water's fine) – at your desk, in the car, on your bedside table – and, if you can, just sip throughout the day. I find that hard to remember, so I drink half a litre (a pint) of water three or four times a day: one before I get out of bed in the morning, another during the morning, another with lunch and another at supper. The amount of fluid you need during training will vary according to the time, the temperature and the intensity of each workout, but should be added on top of your basic daily needs of around two litres (6–8 large glasses). It should be sufficient to prevent you feeling thirsty, and to ensure you produce plenty of pale, straw-coloured urine.

Increase your 'good' calorie intake by experimenting with different fruit and vegetable smoothies and juices, rather than cans of fizzy drink. Test out some caffeine-free hot drinks like redbush, herbal or green tea and try to limit regular tea and coffee to one or two cups a day. It goes without saying that alcohol impairs your general performance in many ways, but I take a relaxed view on this: 'Everything in moderation' leads to a happy athlete!

3. Don't train on empty

Try to plan your training sessions so that you can eat at least one to two hours before setting off. Aim for something that is low in fat, high in carbohydrate, easy to digest and that will gradually release energy to your muscles – a bowl of unrefined porridge, a handful of nuts and raisins and a banana, some fruit and nut muesli with blueberries or a wholemeal sandwich with hummus and rocket. The night before a big workout, make sure you eat a good meal that is rich in slow-burning carbohydrate – spaghetti with parmesan, basil and pine nuts, salmon on saffron rice or a good soup with pulses.

4. Speed up your recovery – eat/drink to refuel within 15 minutes of your long workouts

Carbohydrate is stored in the muscles and liver as glycogen. Glycogen levels become depleted after a workout and the quicker they are topped up again, the quicker your recovery will be and the better you will feel for your next session. You also need water and electrolytes to replace fluid loss, and protein to repair your muscle cells. Grab something as soon as you finish your workout like a honey sandwich, a bowl of rice pudding, a slice of toast with peanut butter or hummus, an energy bar or flapjack, a piece of fruit (melon is good) or a refreshing home-made smoothie made with skimmed milk or yoghurt.

5. Eat well on rest days

Rest days are highly important for recovery as this is the time when your muscles are at their most receptive. For me, it is when the hunger starts to kick in with a vengeance. Make the most of it, replenish your depleted energy stores and feed your muscles by eating well.

Eat well, train well – top Go Faster tips

- *Training burns calories – listen to your body and eat when you are hungry.*
- *An ideal training diet is high in carbohydrate, low in fat with a good mix of protein, vitamins and minerals.*
- *All foods provide energy (calories), but don't waste time with 'empty' calories – make sure each mouthful is nutritious. Stick to fresh, natural ingredients, 'good' calories if you can, and select any processed foods carefully, checking the label for those lowest in hidden fat and salt.*
- *Drink plenty of fluid throughout the day.*
- *Plan your meals and snacks around your exercise – you won't train well on empty.*
- *Eat and drink immediately after an endurance session.*
- *Recovery is key – eat and drink well on rest days to maintain and repair muscle tissues.*

2 the ultimate training diet

A balanced and varied training diet will provide you with all the nutrients and energy you need to achieve your training goals. If you try to eat a variety of the following food types every day, you should be on the right road to attaining your optimum training diet. Remember to aim for about 60 per cent of your total energy intake from carbohydrate, with the balance made up of approximately 15 per cent from protein, and less than 30 per cent from fat. When you are loading up for an endurance competition such as a marathon or triathlon, the amount of carbohydrate you consume should increase significantly to at least 70 per cent (see page 34).

Love your carbs

No matter what your sport, carbohydrate-rich foods are the optimum fuel for energy and, of course, an essential part of the endurance athlete's diet. Carbohydrates, once digested, are eventually converted into blood glucose and used for energy, or stored as glycogen in the liver and muscle. All carbohydrates are not the same, however. Different carbohydrates serve different purposes and we need to choose our carbohydrates wisely. In chapters three and four you will find a more in-depth discussion on carbohydrates and the different types of carbohydrate athletes should focus on, both to maintain stamina and to help recovery.

The amount and type of carbohydrate your body needs varies according to your size and your level of training, but a general rule of thumb is that when training it should be about two-thirds of your daily calorie intake. Try to include a variety of carbohydrate-rich foods in your diet to optimise your intake of nutrients. Focus on carbohydrates that are also rich in vitamins, minerals and fibre, for instance:

- Cereal grains – rice, wheat, oats, barley, corn, rye and anything made from them, such as wholegrain bread, pasta, breakfast cereals, couscous and polenta
- Starchy fruit and vegetables – bananas, potatoes, sweetcorn, carrots, butternut squash, sweet potatoes, pumpkin and parsnips
- Pulses and beans – baked beans, lentils, chickpeas, butter beans, haricot beans and kidney beans

Unrefined carbohydrates are better for our endurance than refined carbohydrates. **Unrefined carbohydrates**, such as wholegrain bread, unprocessed cereals like whole rolled porridge oats, long grain brown rice, wholewheat pasta, pulses and potatoes, are absorbed more slowly into the body, will keep us going for longer and will help avoid dramatic sugar highs and lows**. Refined carbohydrates**, such as short grain white rice, white bread, cakes, biscuits, confectionery and sugar, and sugary products such as sports drinks, are more rapidly absorbed by the body and provide a quick blood sugar rush – great for during or immediately after exercise to replenish tired muscles, but not so good for keeping your energy levels constant on an endurance run.

Go Faster carb tips

- *Base all your meals on carbohydrates.*
- *Don't skip breakfast – try to have something unrefined like porridge made with whole rolled oats, good quality muesli or tomatoes on wholegrain toast. Use brown sugar or, better still, honey, dried fruit or bananas to sweeten your cereal.*
- *Eat carbohydrate-rich snacks – bananas, wholegrain sandwiches, flapjacks, baked beans, dried fruit, malt loaf, scones, teacakes or crumpets.*
- *Remember that pulses are a great source of slow-burning carbohydrate – try soups made with pulses, snacks like falafel and hummus, and add pulses such as chickpeas and butter beans to couscous dishes or stews.*
- *Lentils are a great source of slow-burning energy – they are quick to cook and you don't have to soak them overnight.*
- *There are hundreds of different types of pasta and rice on the supermarket shelves – have fun experimenting with them.*

Eat lots of fruit and vegetables

When you are training hard, your body needs to be well stocked with vitamins and minerals to help you release energy from foods and boost your immune system. Variety is of course the spice of life, so try to include a 'rainbow-coloured' selection of the following different fruit and vegetables in your diet every day for antioxidants including beta-carotene, vitamin C, fibre and folic acid:

- Citrus fruits and berries (for vitamin C and to boost your immune system)
- Greens – spinach, cabbage, watercress, broccoli, fresh herbs (to keep up your iron and folic acid levels and to keep your brain functioning well)

- Brightly coloured fruit or vegetables – carrots, yellow peppers, tomatoes, sweet potatoes, squash (for antioxidants, beta-carotene and vitamin C)

Go Faster fruit and veg tips

- *Drink fresh juices and smoothies to up your fruit and veg intake.*
- *Include fresh fruit with your breakfast every day.*
- *Add loads of delicious fresh herbs to your cooking.*
- *Keep cooking to a minimum – it takes away some of the vitamins (steaming, microwaving and stir-frying are good)*
- *Snack on raw fruit and veg when you are hungry – a carrot, a punnet of blueberries, a nice crunchy apple.*
- *Make exciting salsas with avocados, cucumber, mangoes, fresh herbs and lime juice.*
- *Keep packs of berries in your freezer for puddings.*
- *Make quick, healthy soups using, for instance, watercress, spinach or carrot to start your meal.*
- *Have a portion of fresh veg or a salad with every meal. Don't forget that frozen and canned fruit and veg also count towards your five portions a day.*

Protein for power and recovery

Meat, fish and alternatives

Our bodies need a certain amount of meat, fish or vegetarian alternatives such as eggs, cheese, nuts or pulses to ensure that we get enough iron, protein, zinc, magnesium and B vitamins. Your body will often need extra protein after an event or a heavy training session to help repair damage to the muscles. This might be why so many people crave a nice juicy steak after a competition. Try to include a couple of servings per day from the following selection in your diet:

- Lean meat
- Fish and shellfish
- Eggs or cheese
- Pulses, Quorn, beans or pulses such as soya or soya bean curd (tofu) are great alternatives if you are vegetarian
- Beans, nuts and dark chocolate to keep your immune system functioning well

Go Faster protein tips

- *Include poultry or fish a couple of times a week as a healthy alternative to red meat.*
- *Cook meat and fish on a griddle or grill to reduce fat content.*
- *Red meats such as lean steak, lean mince, and offal such as liver, along with delicious treats like venison, calves' liver, clams, mussels, scallops and oysters are really high in easily absorbed iron. Pulses and beans contain plant versions of iron, which is less easily absorbed, but you can eat vitamin C (e.g. tomatoes, broccoli, orange juice) with these foods, which will help your body absorb this type of iron.*
- *Snack on nuts or sprinkle roasted nuts onto breakfast cereals, salads or couscous.*

Don't forget milk and dairy products or non-dairy alternatives

If you are taking regular and vigorous exercise you need to make sure your body is getting enough calcium. Milk and dairy foods provide this, along with protein, vitamins A and B12 and riboflavin (which helps release energy from carbohydrates), and are important for the health of our bones, skin and blood. Try to have a couple of decent helpings of milk, cheese or yoghurt every day. If you are lactose intolerant there are plenty of calcium-fortified non-dairy alternatives, such as soya-based products, available and, of course, you can top up your calcium levels with pulses, green, leafy vegetables (such as broccoli or kale), and oily fish and nuts (almonds are particularly good).

Go Faster calcium tips

- *If you don't like milk, try to replace it with yoghurt or calcium-fortified soya milk.*
- *Use natural yoghurt and fromage frais in sauces and salad dressings.*
- *Use low-fat versions if you feel this is necessary.*
- *My favourite way of increasing dairy intake is to use lots of parmesan cheese on my risottos, pasta and salads.*
- *Grilled haloumi cheese with a sweet chilli sauce is a hit with the kids, even the ones who do not like cheese.*
- *Don't obsess about cutting out saturated fats like cream and butter, but do use them in moderation and avoid the obvious 'no-nos' like very creamy pasta sauces, slabs of butter on your toast or large dollops of clotted cream on your apple crumble. It is difficult to get 60 per cent plus of your calories from carbohydrates if you eat a lot of fat, so you would be wise to cut down if your diet is high in fat, especially saturated fat.*

Some oils and fats are good

There are three main types of fat: saturated, monounsaturated and polyunsaturated. Most foods contain a mixture. Unsaturated fats – omega-3 and omega-6 – are actually good for us. These are the fats found in oily fish, nuts and seeds and cold-pressed vegetable oils, and they should be an essential part of our diet. They can reduce the risk of cardiovascular disease, and may even play a role in improving your mood and brain power. Saturated fats, on the other hand, such as butter, the juicy bit of fat on your steak, the crackling on your roast pork, and hydrogenated vegetable oils found in processed foods such as pastry, cakes and biscuits, should be kept to a reasonable minimum.

Go Faster fat tips

- *Treat yourself to oily fish such as mackerel, salmon, pilchards, sardines or fresh tuna once a week for omega-3 content. Grilled tinned sardines or mackerel on toast make a great lunch (although fresh is even more delicious!).*
- *Buy packs of seeds for snacks and sprinkle sunflower and pumpkin seeds on your cereal.*
- *Roast your own nuts and use them in your cooking – walnuts in salads, pine nuts on pasta, and pistachios with couscous.*
- *Experiment with different oils. Use olive oil instead of butter (for example, in mashed potatoes and for cooking), try delicious pumpkin seed oil in salad dressings and cold-pressed rapeseed oil for frying – it is rich in vitamin E and omega-3 and heats to a really high temperature without losing its nutrients, to give excellent crispy results.*

Go faster 'rainbow' superfoods

Beyond the basic food classifications – protein, fat and carbohydrates, fibre, vitamins and essential minerals – a new unofficial food category has recently emerged which can be loosely classed as 'superfoods', or 'rainbow foods'. These are foods that contain phytonutrients (plant-derived essential nutrients). Phytonutrients are usually related to the colour of the food, hence the term 'rainbow foods', with different colours containing different nutrients, for example lycopene in tomatoes, carotenoids in yellow, orange and red fruit and vegetables, and flavonoids in blueberries. Phytonutrients are said to have medicinal properties which support the immune system, help prevent a variety of diseases and can help carry out the metabolic processes that actually produce energy. That may be true, but for me the brilliant thing about these superfoods is that they are healthy *and* exceedingly delicious – really worth including in your training diet. What's more, they don't have to be expensive – many basic fruit and vegetables, seeds, nuts, pulses and wholegrains can be reasonably classed as superfoods.

Of course, no food is 'super' unless it is eaten as part of a balanced and varied diet – pigging out on ten punnets of blueberries will bankrupt you and won't make you any healthier in the long run as your body can only absorb and store a certain amount of each nutrient. However, including a rainbow of these different coloured superfoods in a balanced, varied and unprocessed diet should set you on the right path towards the perfect 'super' training diet.

Go Faster Superfoods

- *apricots – dried*
- *artichokes*
- *avocados*
- *bananas*
- *berries – blueberries, cranberries, raspberries, strawberries etc*
- *chilli peppers*
- *citrus fruits*
- *cocoa*
- *garlic*
- *green tea, redbush tea and other herbal teas*
- *green, yellow, red and orange fruit – apples, peaches, apricots, kiwis, mangoes, melons, squash, yam, carrots, pumpkin, pomegranate, sweet potato, watermelon*
- *leafy greens – cabbage, Brussels sprouts, cauliflower, spinach, broccoli*
- *nuts – almonds, Brazils, walnuts etc*
- *oily fish*
- *olive oil, rapeseed oil, pumpkin seed oil*
- *onions*
- *porridge oats*
- *pulses – beans, peas, lentils*
- *red/green/yellow peppers*
- *red wine*
- *seeds – sunflower seeds, flax seeds, sesame seeds, pumpkin seeds*
- *soy beans*
- *tomatoes*
- *wholegrain wheat, oats, barley or rye*

3 get your carbs right:

carbohydrates and the glycaemic index (G.I.)

Carbohydrate – why so important?

No matter what your sport, carbohydrate-rich foods are critical for optimum performance – so critical that they deserve a whole chapter devoted to them. Our muscles depend on carbohydrate as their main source of fuel for exercise. Carbohydrate is digested and then absorbed into the body as blood glucose. It is either used or stored as glycogen in the liver and muscle for later use. If our glycogen levels are low, fatigue sets in, our stamina begins to wane, we lose concentration and our performance is impaired. What is more, our recovery becomes less efficient.

The amount of carbohydrate that our bodies are able to store as glycogen in the liver and muscles is really quite small. Regular intense training quickly depletes these small reserves and this is why it is so essential to eat a substantial amount of carbohydrate every day to maximise our energy stores. If we do not keep our glycogen stores topped up the body starts to manufacture glucose from muscle protein instead. Deriving energy from fat uses much more oxygen and taking energy from muscle protein eventually leads to loss of muscle mass and consequently strength – not good news for an endurance athlete.

Even when we carbo-load before a race, the limited amount our bodies can store is used up after a couple of hours of continuous intensive exercise, so we start to draw on the energy stores in our fat and muscles instead. This is when we start to get extremely tired and 'hit the wall'. In these situations we must learn to build up our starting stores and restock our system with a form of carbohydrate that we can digest rapidly.

In short, carbohydrates play an essential role before, during and after exercise – a low-carb diet is an unwise choice for an endurance athlete.

The right carb at the right time – it makes all the difference

All carbohydrates are not equal, however, as they all break down to glucose at different rates. In 1981, Dr David Jenkins, a professor in the Department of Nutritional Sciences at the University of Toronto, developed a method of classifying carbohydrates to indicate the speed at which they release sugars into the bloodstream. This is referred to as the Glycaemic Index, or G.I. in which carbohydrate-rich foods are given a G.I. rating between 0 and 100.

Fast-acting High-G.I. Carbs (G.I. of 70 or more) – to reach our muscles fast

High-G.I. carbohydrates (such as sugar, some rice, baked potatoes and cornflakes) break down quickly during digestion and are absorbed more quickly into the bloodstream, resulting in a surge of blood glucose. A high-G.I. drink or snack just before or during sport gives your muscles a quick energy boost. Likewise, the body resynthesises glycogen at a faster rate immediately after exercise, so consuming high G.I. carbohydrates straight after endurance will increase the rate at which our muscles can recover and gives us the stamina to continue training. A honey sandwich made with white bread, for instance, eaten immediately after a long run, followed by a good broad bean risotto once you have summoned up enough energy to cook, is a great way to get high G.I. carbohydrate quickly into your system.

If you regularly eat large amounts of high-G.I. foods, your body can produce too much insulin, the hormone which metabolises the carbohydrate and transports it to the liver and muscles. This causes hunger pangs and energy slumps. Therefore, you should try to limit high-G.I. carbohydrates to immediately before and after exercise and concentrate on low- to medium-G.I. carbohydrates for your regular diet.

Slower-burning Low- to Medium-G.I. Carbs (G.I. of 70 and below) – for sustained energy

Low- to medium-G.I. carbohydrates (pasta, pulses, oats, most fruit and veg) break down slowly during digestion, releasing glucose more gradually into the bloodstream thus maintaining a much more stable level of blood glucose. The lower the G.I., the slower the rate of digestion and, therefore, the more gradual the supply of energy to the muscles. If your carbohydrate intake is predominantly made up of low- to medium-G.I. foods, you will find that you will not get hungry so quickly and your energy levels will increase and be more sustained. You will have more stamina and training will become easier. A low- to medium-G.I. meal at least two to three hours before a workout will delay fatigue, as energy will be transported to the muscles more gradually and prolong the time before that dreaded exhaustion sets in.

The Simple Go Faster Carb Rules

- Think low- to medium-G.I. carbohydrate foods for your general training diet, especially the night before or 2–3 hours before long endurance sessions. This will help regulate your blood sugar levels and maintain your energy levels.
- Think high-G.I. carbohydrate foods for immediately before, during and immediately after exercise and for your recovery meal after heavy endurance sessions when you have given your muscles a serious beating. This will give you a surge of energy and help your muscles recover more quickly.

These simple rules are particularly important as you reach the peak levels of your training. You may be running over 40 miles a week if you are training for a marathon, for instance, or doing 9–10 hours swimming, cycling and running a week if you are training for a half-ironman. At this point most people find that they are so incredibly hungry *all* the time that they are eating like a bear before hibernation. I personally find that I am even more ravenous on my rest days as my body is fighting to catch up on all those calories I have burnt.

High G.I. or Low G.I. – how can I tell the difference?

Here is a list of common low-, medium- and high-G.I. foods. Note that, if you combine high- and low-G.I. foods, the effect of the high-G.I. food is reduced. For instance, adding low-G.I. semi-skimmed milk to a high-G.I. bowl of cornflakes makes it a medium-G.I. meal.

Low-G.I. foods – G.I. of 0–55

- *Porridge*
- *Muesli (no sugar)*
- *Oat cereals*
- *High-fibre bran such as All-Bran™*
- *Spaghetti and most fresh and dried pasta*
- *Egg noodles*
- *Glass noodles*
- *Pumpernickel bread*
- *Granary/stoneground wholemeal/sourdough bread*
- *Wholemeal pitta bread*
- *Pulses such as lentils and chickpeas*
- *Beans such as kidney, mung, soya, haricot, butter, blackeye, borlotti and baked beans*
- *Bulgur wheat*
- *Most dairy products – milk, cream, natural yoghurt, cottage cheese, hard cheese, ricotta etc*
- *Fruit – apples, citrus fruits, bananas, figs, kiwi, mangoes, red berries, blueberries*

- *Vegetables – broccoli, beansprouts, cauliflower, green beans, leafy greens, aubergines, avocado, salad vegetables such as lettuce, rocket and watercress, cabbage, mushrooms, tomatoes*
- *Dried apricots*
- *Nuts and seeds, peanut butter, tahini, hummus*
- *Fruit loaf*
- *Tea, milk drinks (no sugar)*

Medium-G.I. foods – G.I. of 55-70

- *Muesli (with sugar)*
- *Wholewheat cereals*
- *White pitta bread/most brown bread*
- *Crumpets, oatcakes*
- *Couscous*
- *Basmati rice, dried rice noodles*
- *Brown rice, risotto rice*
- *Polenta*
- *Boiled potatoes with skin*
- *Vegetables – beetroot, sweetcorn, peas, carrots, sweet potatoes*
- *Fruit – fresh pineapple, melon, apricots, canned fruits*
- *Dried sultanas, raisins, prunes*
- *Muffins – bran, blueberry, banana*
- *Honey, jam and marmalade*

High-G.I. foods – G.I. of 70 and above

- *Processed cereals such as bran flakes, Cornflakes, puffed rice and sugary cereals*
- *White rice (not basmati)*
- *Rice pudding*
- *White bread, baguette*
- *Bagels, rice cakes, crackers*
- *Potatoes – boiled and peeled, baked, fried, mashed – old potatoes have a higher G.I. than new (because of the type of starch)*
- *Vegetables – broad beans, parsnips, pumpkin, swede, turnip, cassava*
- *Watermelon*
- *Dates*
- *Sports glucose drinks*
- *Hot chocolate/cocoa*
- *Jelly beans*
- *Many processed fast foods such as burgers and pizzas*

4 top go faster carbs

Oats

Oats really are the ultimate grain for the athlete's breakfast. They have a low glycaemic index and a high percentage of carbohydrate and fibre. They can also help lower cholesterol and maintain a healthy digestive system. Most importantly, however, they keep you going for ages. Unrefined, whole rolled Scottish jumbo porridge oats are the tastiest and the most sustaining and are fantastic in porridge, muesli and flapjacks. You can usually find them in the supermarket on the same shelf as the quick-cook varieties, which have a slightly higher G.I. and are less effective for endurance.

Many people find that a pre-workout bowl of porridge made with water rather than milk is better for the digestion. Milk can irritate the stomach and play havoc with the digestive system, particularly if you are feeling nervous.

'Best pre-race breakfast? Porridge with banana, nuts and seeds, and some eggs.' Oli Beckingsale, professional cyclist. Cross-country mountain bike: three times Olympian, Commonwealth silver, five times National Senior Champion.

Pasta

'My mum makes me pesto pasta with extra pine nuts and bacon on race days. I snack on it throughout the day, even at the poolside before I race.' Oliver Eyre, swimmer. National Swimming Championships 2007, 100m, 200m and 400m freestyle.

Normal wheat pasta of any shape, fresh or dried, is a fabulous food for athletes. It has a low glycaemic index (30–50), it is low in fat and extremely high in carbohydrate. There are endless possibilities for cooking this fabulous, sustaining food, just as there are hundreds of different pasta varieties available – you can put the old staple Spaghetti Bolognese on the back burner if you want (although it really is very tasty and will always be one of my favourites). Fresh pasta makes a wonderfully delicious fast food – I guarantee it is quicker, and a whole lot healthier, to knock up a bowl of fresh pasta than it is to wait for any take-away. The wholewheat variety contains more fibre, minerals (manganese, magnesium, iron) and B vitamins than its white counterpart, so it is good to include this in your training diet.

Rice

Rice also has a high percentage of carbohydrate and has for a long time been regarded as a great fuel for athletes. Rice is low in fat and is an excellent source of vitamin E, B vitamins (thiamin and niacin) and potassium. Rice is usually classified by the size of grain, the most common types being long-grain (long and slender, for instance basmati), medium-grain (shorter and plumper, like paella or risotto rice) and short-grain (for instance pudding rice). A basic rule is, the longer the grain, the lower the G.I.

White rice

White rice is pretty bland in taste and is great with spicy foods, such as Thai or Indian food. However, the bran and the germ have been removed which means that a lot of the nutrients are lost. White rice (apart from basmati rice) has a high G.I. factor and so is an excellent food to eat after a big endurance session. Try Thai fragrant jasmine rice with your curry or, if you want to use a rice with a really high G.I., then go for a delicious and comforting rice pudding made with pudding rice or glutinous rice.

Basmati rice

Both white and brown basmati rice have the lowest G.I. factor (58) out of all the different varieties of rice, and make a perfect staple for an athlete's diet. I use this rice in my general cooking as it tends to be deliciously light and fluffy, versatile, easy to prepare and easy to digest.

'Favourite meal the night before an event? Fish, brown rice, red peppers, broccoli, peas.' Andy Wadsworth, fitness consultant, personal trainer, mountain biker and world-class triathlete. Xterra Triathlon World Champion.

Brown rice

Brown rice really is a much better source of B vitamins, minerals and fibre than white rice. It does take longer to cook, although it is now possible to buy quicker-cooking brown basmati rice in the supermarkets. It has a lovely nutty flavour and it is very filling. Brown basmati is an exceptionally good sustaining food to eat the night before a race.

Risotto rice

Risotto rice has a G.I. factor of 69, at the highest end of the medium-G.I. category. My family loves risottos and I find them a very useful medium for disguising whatever might be lurking in the fridge and at the back of the cupboard or vegetable rack – a tin of artichokes or a butternut squash, for instance – without anyone realising. I tend to cook a lot of risottos when we are training, especially for evenings after a big workout; they are comforting on the stomach and make for a good night's sleep. You need to stand over the risotto to stir it for about 20 minutes: a wonderful excuse to switch off, listen to the radio and do your stretches.

Rice noodles

Cellophane rice noodles are the ultimate fast food carbohydrate. They have a low G.I. and are very quick and easy to prepare – generally you just need to pour boiling water over them and wait for about three minutes. They are very useful for adding to oriental soups or for eating with Thai curries.

Other varieties of rice

Try experimenting with different types of speciality rice. Good ones to try are wild rice (good to mix with basmati), three-grain rice, Spanish paella rice, red Camargue rice and black pudding rice.

Couscous and Bulgur Wheat

Couscous is one of my favourite carbohydrates. It is extremely versatile, a doddle to make and very, very tasty. With a medium G.I. of 68, it provides a good source of carbohydrate, especially when eaten with other low-G.I. foods such as chickpeas, and it contains high levels of fibre, B vitamins and iron. Couscous is also quite light on the stomach, easy to digest and not too filling, so you can eat a substantial amount of it at any one time.

Couscous is made from 100 per cent durum wheat flour and is light and fluffy. It is traditionally served plain with a tagine (middle-eastern stew) or a kebab, but you can use it to make salads, serve it warm with roasted vegetables, herbs and spices, and bulk it up with pulses – the possibilities are endless. If you are lucky enough to have children who will eat couscous, it makes a great quick and nutritious family meal; just pour boiling water or stock over the couscous, stir and wait for 5–10 minutes.

Bulgur wheat has a lower G.I. than couscous (48) and a delicious nutty flavour. It releases carbohydrate into your bloodstream nice and slowly and it is a good source of fibre, thiamin, vitamin E and minerals. It is more substantial than couscous, so not quite as light, but it is really good in Tabbouleh, a traditional Middle Eastern herb salad.

A couscous or a bulgur wheat salad is a very good midday meal if you are planning a gym session or a tempo run in the early evening. I often make too much so that I can keep some in the fridge for a lunchbox or to snack on when I am feeling peckish.

As couscous has a medium G.I. rather than a low one, I would usually add some low-G.I. pulses to it (a can of chickpeas for instance) if I want my meal to help towards a big endurance session. Some people find pasta a little too heavy for a pre-race meal – couscous can make a good alternative.

Polenta

Polenta is a lovely way of eating carbohydrate as part of your training diet and makes a great substitute for rice and pasta. It has a medium G.I., it is low in fat, high in carbohydrate and is very easy to digest. The instant variety is really quick to cook; the traditional variety takes a little longer, and of course is all the more delicious for it. Made from cornmeal, polenta has a smooth, creamy texture but a bland taste if you cook it with water alone. Once you add some herbs, plenty of freshly ground black pepper and some tasty olive oil, it is really quite delicious. You can cook it as soft polenta or you can cook it for a little longer and leave it to cool and then cut it into slices to be fried or grilled.

Gnocchi

Gnocchi are little Italian dumplings, usually made from flour and potato, bound together with egg. They are delicious with a simple tomato or pesto sauce and are good to eat as a recovery food as they contain a little protein as well as carbohydrate. They take only a few minutes to cook, especially if you use the ready-made fresh gnocchi which are available in most supermarkets. If you are feeling adventurous, try making them yourself (see page 175).

Lentils and Pulses

Most lentils and pulses have a G.I. of less than 50. They are slow-releasing, low in fat and extremely nutritious. They can help lower cholesterol and are rich in carbohydrate, protein, B vitamins, fibre and minerals such as iron, calcium and zinc. They are also said to increase immunity levels and help towards reducing the risk of certain cancers. I find that they really help to sustain you and I try to include them in my training diet as much as possible, even if it means just adding a tin of chickpeas to my favourite sauce or casserole.

Many varieties of beans need to be soaked overnight before you use them. I think they taste better than the tinned varieties, but by all means use these to save time as they are still full of goodness.

Potatoes

Although packed with nutrition, potatoes always come second place to pasta and rice owing to their lower percentage of carbohydrate. They also tend to be on the higher end of the G.I. spectrum – boiled new potatoes, unpeeled, have a lower G.I. than mashed, baked and chipped, which have a G.I. of 80–85. Potatoes are good to include in your training diet, however, as they contain good quantities of vitamin C, along with potassium, iron, fibre and other minerals. You can lower the G.I. by mixing your potatoes with a lower G.I. food, such as baked beans on a jacket potato.

5

what to eat and when – putting theory into practice

Fuel-up your training

Eating the right foods is all very well in theory, but the practice can be so very different. When you are planning your exercise around a busy work schedule or around family commitments, it is hard enough getting the exercise in, let alone buying, preparing and eating the correct food at the correct time. Not only do you have to plan carefully when you are going to exercise, you also have to plan when you are going to eat. Sometimes I get this completely wrong – I am either not hungry enough to face eating before an early morning run, or I am too ravenous to even consider doing any exercise in the evening.

It is very difficult to get it right all the time.

Sometimes you have to leave so early in the morning for a race that it's an uphill struggle to eat enough. My worst experience of this was the early start before the New York Marathon. At 5am, we were desperately trying to force down our porridge so that we could be in line at the bus stop by 6am to get over the Verrazano-Narrows Bridge before it closed at 7am, even though the start was hours later at 10am. By this time, the energy from the little porridge I had managed to eat had been used up and I was relying on flapjacks, gels and sports drink – not a great combination for an already nervous stomach!

Of course, what you eat on the day and during the week leading up to a competition is crucial, but it really is what you eat on a daily basis during your training that will have the greatest impact. It will help you train better, which in turn will produce your best performance on race day.

Practical Go Faster fuelling tips

- *Plan ahead – think about when and how intensively you will be training, and time your meals and snacks to fit in with this.*
- *Keep your cupboards well stocked (see page 272).*
- *Cook larger quantities of meals like soups and stews and store portions in the freezer – remove from the freezer to defrost in the morning and when you get home, all you need to do is reheat.*
- *If possible, shop on a daily basis for small amounts of fresh ingredients.*

Exercising at sunrise

If you like to train early in the morning, you should try your best to fuel up before you exercise, especially if you are doing a session of 40 minutes or longer. You will not have eaten anything for about 10 hours, your blood sugar and insulin levels will be low and so it stands to reason that your body and brain will not function at their optimum level without some sustenance.

If you can, get up an hour before you exercise and drink a big glass of water as soon as you wake up. Leave dressing and getting ready until after you have eaten breakfast to give yourself the maximum time to digest. If you are planning a long session, try a high-carbohydrate power breakfast, like porridge with honey and sunflower seeds, fruit and nut muesli with blueberries, or Birchermuesli. Birchermuesli (see page 58) is a great option as you will have prepared it the night before and it will be just sitting in the fridge waiting to be eaten.

This approach is not always practical, especially if you are one of those people who cannot face getting out from under that nice, warm duvet until the last possible moment. I find that anything I consume within an hour of exercise plays havoc with my stomach and impairs my running ability – half a banana and a glucose tablet or half a slice of toast is about all I can manage. The only thing you can do is try your best to fuel up the night before with a high-carbohydrate, low- to medium-G.I. meal, like a bowl of spaghetti with basil, pine nuts and parmesan (see page 112) or lemon and fennel pilaf with garlic prawns (see page 161). You will find your performance and endurance will be a lot better if you have eaten this rather than take-away fish and chips, for instance.

You return from your early morning session, shower quickly, dress and rush straight off to work, to do the school run or maybe both. Try your best to take a few extra minutes to eat something so that you avoid those 11 o'clock hunger pangs and that overwhelming feeling of fatigue halfway through the day – whack some fruit into the blender for a smoothie or toast a couple of slices of wholegrain bread and boil yourself an egg.

Lunchtime workouts

Exercising at lunchtime means that you have plenty of time to fuel up. Unless you have had an extremely late breakfast, your blood sugar will have dipped and you will feel so hungry by the time you want to exercise that you will be tempted to skip your workout. Try to eat a pre-lunch snack about one hour or so beforehand. If you are at work, take in an energy-giving hummus and rocket sandwich, a flapjack (see page 227) or a big slice of Go Faster carrot cake (see page 244).

Eat some lunch after your exercise or you will find that by 4 o'clock you will have completely run out of steam. Try something quick and easy to eat, like a bowl of soup with bread or some cous-cous salad.

Evening stress-busting

Exercising in the evening is a great stress-buster. The problem is that you often feel too lethargic or too ravenous to face it. This is usually because you have not eaten or drunk enough during the day. If you want to exercise in the evening, make sure you have a good breakfast and a proper lunch. Grab a mid-afternoon snack and drink plenty of water throughout the day. After your exercise, try your best to have a decent evening meal or you may find it difficult to sleep – there is nothing worse than lying in bed with an empty stomach. If you can, it is best to exercise early in the evening, as the later you leave it, the harder it will be to fit in a proper meal, and to get to sleep. My husband has a very energetic game of tennis with friends twice a week, starting at 8.30pm. This plays havoc with sleep and digestion if he gets the timing wrong. He finds that the best solution is to eat a meal, or at least a sandwich, at about 6.30pm in preparation. This keeps the wolf from the door for the evening. If he needs something afterwards, he tries to limit it to a small snack, such as a bowl of cereal.

Recovery and the importance of eating well on rest days

We all know that it is crucial to eat well during training, but remember that rest days are just as important as workout days. Your body not only needs to recover from the previous day, but energy levels must also be topped up for the following days' endurance. It can take up to 20 hours for muscle glycogen stores to be fully replenished after a heavy workout, as glycogen is restored to the muscles at a rate of 5 per cent per hour. Training intensely on a regular basis means that you need to recover from the previous session, that is, your body's glycogen stores need to be replenished as quickly as possible, so that you can start again on the next. If you fail to refuel properly over a period of time, the glycogen reserves in your working muscles will become progressively depleted – you will feel lethargic and your muscles will feel heavy and tired. Maintaining your carb-rich diet on rest days, you will delay the onset of fatigue and help avoid those dreadful days when your legs feel like lumps of lead.

The amount of carbohydrate you need for recovery varies according to your weight and the intensity of your workout. These are the guidelines recommended by the International Olympic Committee Consensus Statement on Sports Nutrition (2004):

Type of training	Carbohydrate requirements for daily recovery (g carbohydrate/kg body weight per day)
Moderate duration/low intensity	*5–7g*
Moderate to heavy endurance training	*7–12g*
Extreme exercise programmes (> 4–6 hours per day)	*10–12g*

Gearing up for a competition

The week before

What you eat and drink during the week before a competition can have an enormous effect on your performance. It is generally accepted practice nowadays to taper training during the week prior to a race and to increase the intake of carbohydrate and fluid, so that glycogen levels are as high as possible. In practical terms, this means that you should reduce your training to decrease the use of muscle glycogen whilst eating your normal high-carbohydrate diet up until the last three days before the race. You should then increase the carbohydrate content of your diet to about 70 per cent. You should aim to consume about 8–10g of carbohydrate per kg of body weight – if you weigh 65kg, aim for between 520g and 650g per day; if you weigh 80kg, aim for between 640g and 800g per day. Don't get too hung up on data, just slightly increase the amount of carbs in your already high-carb diet and decrease the amount of protein. Take a look at the menu plans on page 263 to give you some idea of what you could be eating.

Examples of foods and drinks containing 50g of carbohydrate

Foods

2 large bananas or 3 apples, oranges or pears
3 slices thick sliced bread or 1 bagel
2–3 slices malt loaf
1 large bowl breakfast cereal
4 tablespoons cooked rice
8 tablespoons cooked pasta (200g)
75g noodles (1 sheet)
1 medium jacket potato
1 can baked beans (400g)
15 dried apricots
2 cereal bars

Drinks

1 litre semi-skimmed milk
500ml fruit juice
800ml isotonic sports drink
330ml fruit smoothie

Drink copiously during this week (water, not alcohol!) to get your body really well hydrated. Aim for about three litres a day.

The day before

You should really rest or do a little light exercise the day before. Don't make the mistake my husband made (although, it has to be said, under my very bad influence) the first time he ran a marathon in New York. Carried away by the excitement of being in New York, we spent the day before seeing as many sights as possible – China

Town, Greenwich Village, Central Park, Wall Street ... We must have walked about 12 miles through the streets of Manhattan. It was the worst preparation possible for his legs.

As regards to food, it is best to stick to what you are familiar with the day before an endurance event. Don't try anything new, avoid high fat, indigestible foods and choose a good plain lunch and supper. Eat enough to ensure that your body is well-fuelled but don't overeat or you will not sleep well. You need to do this, as you may feel too nervous the next day to get much down you. My favourites are spaghetti with basil, pine nuts and parmesan and spaghetti with fresh herbs. Both contain a high percentage of low-G.I. carbohydrate, plus a few vitamins, a little protein and not too much fibre. Avoid alcohol or keep it to the very minimum and drink lots of water during the day, but be careful to stop quite early so that you are not plagued by loo visits during the night.

Race morning!

'It's better to be overnourished (and more fun) than undernourished for races ... get enough fuel in the tank to finish strong ... make sure it is properly digested and does not sit in the stomach.' Michelle Lee, triathlete, marathoner, cyclist, duathlete, professional sportsperson, teacher, mum, sport and remedial massage therapist. World Duathlon 2006–08 (3rd); marathon personal best: 2:35.

Eat your pre-competition breakfast about 2–3 hours before the start time. Again, eat and drink something that you are familiar with, and don't try anything new. If you are doing a distance event, for instance a distance triathlon, it is best to eat as late as possible – up to 90 minutes before the event – as you will need to keep enough in the tank for the latter part of the race.

Stick to what you have eaten and drunk during your training 'dress rehearsal'. If you are away from home, ask the hotel or bed and breakfast to make up your favourite breakfast – I know several athletes, including myself, who have resorted to preparing porridge in the hotel room to avoid the continental breakfast on offer in the hotel dining room – it is not really a race preparation to be recommended.

Think about your drinking strategy as toilet facilities for different events can really vary. I try to drink about ½ litre of water approximately three hours before the race and then just sip on a sports drink at regular intervals until the start.

If the event is in the afternoon, eat a really good breakfast and then have a light, easy-to-digest lunch – spaghetti with tomato sauce, for instance.

Take a snack with you to have in the start area while you are waiting. I do find it difficult to eat just before a race, but if you can stomach it, it is worth it. I usually take a honey sandwich or a flapjack and normally manage a few bites. If you are too nervous, then stick to a sports drink.

Of course, you could ignore all this advice and survive on adrenalin to a certain point, as my 15-year-old daughter did before her first ever sprint triathlon last year. She was so nervous, it was as much as I could do to get a few bites of cereal and a nibble of her favourite flapjack down her before the race. The sea swim went brilliantly, despite the heavy current, and the cycling was absolutely fine, but as she started the run the adrenalin petered out and she, my normally gazelle-like girl, plodded her way through to the finish line like a tortoise.

During the race

'The biggest issues whilst training [for the Marathon des Sables] were eating and drinking on the move, both of which I found challenging due to stitches and feeling sick! On the event we had to carry 2,500 calories for each day and it needed to be as light as possible. My final food consisted of granola cereal and nuts for breakfast, and throughout the day I would snack on flapjacks, granola bars, nuts (nice and salty), biltong (I'm miserable without protein), jelly babies (quick sugar burst and morale boost!) and salt tablets. Supper was a freeze-dried meal. I would always eat breakfast and supper but was appalling at eating throughout the day – the elite runner in our tent gobbled up everyone's leftovers each night.' Vicky Ryan, teacher, head of girls' games, marathon runner and member of the England mixed touch rugby. Completed the Marathon des Sables (a six-day, 220km endurance race across the Sahara Desert) in 2006.

Your performance and endurance can be enhanced with extra carbohydrate during the race, especially if you are taking part in an event lasting over 90 minutes. It is important to find out what suits you as an individual, so try different strategies during your training. You may surprise yourself that you can actually eat something solid to keep you going – a banana or a piece of malt loaf, for instance, or you may find that you can only manage a carbohydrate sports drink or a handful of jelly babies. Again, see the menu plans on page 263 for suitable choices.

Post-race

It is important to refuel and rehydrate as quickly as possible after an event. The same rules apply as after long training sessions, so try to eat a high-G.I. snack within 15 minutes of finishing and gulp down a carbohydrate sports drink. It might be the last thing you fancy doing, but it really does speed up your recovery. Aim to consume 1–1.2g of carbohydrate per kg of body weight per hour over the four hours after an endurance race (or endurance training session) to help recovery.

There is often a bar at the finish line of certain events – in fact there were several beer stands at the finishers' area of the Berlin Marathon. Find the willpower to ignore these, drink plenty of water, and wait until your body has readjusted itself a little before you have that celebratory drink or you will feel gruesome the next day. Have a delicious post-event meal as soon as you can and make sure it is balanced. It needs to be high in high-G.I. carbohydrate with a decent amount of protein and minerals – a good risotto, or a mild Thai curry with jasmine rice, for instance.

You will find that you will be ravenous for a good few days. Your metabolic rate will still be racing, so listen to your body, rest and enjoy yourself with some great food and drink – you deserve it! Remember the old Chinese proverb: 'When the belly is full, the bones are at rest'.

Favourite post-race meals

'I'm afraid this isn't going to look pretty. It'll always include at least 500g of chocolate, several cakes and a pizza or three.' Adam Bardsley, Managing Director, Ironman (personal best: 10:28) and marathon (personal best: 2:41) runner. Completed Ironman France 2008.

'There is nothing better than a glass of red wine and a good meal ... followed by a hot, relaxing bath.' Mavis Paterson a.k.a. Grannymave, 70, retired nurse, long-distance cyclist and runner. Completed 4,500 mile transcontinental bike ride across Canada, 2008.

'Pizza and chocolate! Anytime, anyplace, anywhere!' Michelle Lee, triathlete, marathoner, cyclist, duathlete, professional sportsperson, teacher, mum, sport and remedial massage therapist. World Duathlon 2006–08 (3rd); marathon personal best: 2:35.

'Usually I feel the need for a good protein meal, for example steak.' Carolyn Forsyth, housewife, mother of three and marathon runner (personal best: 3:13). Completed Davos Alpine Marathon.

'It has to be steak and chips!' Mark Collingwood, solicitor and marathon runner (personal best: 3:24). Best event – Amsterdam Marathon 2006.

'Steak and chips and a beer always hits the spot.' Oli Beckingsale, professional cyclist. Cross country mountain bike: three times Olympian, Commonwealth Silver, five times National Senior Champion.

'Cold beer – you deserve it! Anything on offer. Pasta, chips, omelettes, anything goes. Did I mention the cold beer?' Adam Mason, TV sports rights manager, runner, cyclist, swimmer and skier. Best event – Étape du Tour 2007.

6

hydration, hydration, hydration!

Do you ever feel so exhausted that you have to stop running? Do you sometimes feel dizzy or disorientated during a long workout? Have you ever been overcome by cramp after cycling for 60km?

These are all signs of dehydration rearing its ugly head. Exercise makes us sweat; it is our body's efficient way of trying to maintain a steady temperature. During long periods of intense exercise the loss of large amounts of sweat can not only have a negative effect on our performance, but ignoring symptoms can also lead to serious consequences.

Even the well-conditioned athlete has to be careful about hydration, especially in hot conditions. As the heat increases, so does your core body temperature and you start to sweat profusely. This causes a decrease in your blood volume, which is necessary for carrying oxygen to the heart. Consequently, there is less oxygen-rich blood available to fuel your working muscles – your muscles are being pushed to capacity but they are receiving fewer nutrients and you start to slow down. What is more, on a hot day your body tries to cool itself by sending more blood into the capillaries (small blood vessels) of the skin and the amount of blood available to the muscles is reduced even further. You become increasingly dehydrated as your body fights to maintain its core temperature.

When my very best running buddy collapsed at the finish line of the London Marathon in April 2008, it struck me more than ever that if we are pushing the boundaries of our physical and mental endurance, we really need to be serious about both our diet and drinking strategy – not just to enhance our performance, but also to prevent injury, exhaustion, or even worse. After 30 minutes in the medical tent, my buddy was fully recovered, if a little shaken, having been given a magic glucose drink and some very welcome massage. Digging a little deeper into why this should have happened to a fit, well-trained athlete who had eaten a good training diet, I discovered that in fact he had taken on very little fluid – not only during the race, but also during the week running up to the race. He had been so set on beating his PB (which he missed by eight seconds!) that he had only taken the odd sip of water at the drinks stations, plus a gel at mile six. Had he taken the time to grab a sports drink or an orange segment or two, perhaps he would have made up those vital seconds.

'I have only recently come to terms with the fact that I need to drink more during the race – I tend to get too carried along with the atmosphere and forget.' Mark Collingwood, solicitor, marathon runner (personal best – 3:24). Best event – London Marathon 2006.

Be serious about drinking

Each person has an individual requirement for fluid – body weight, gender, climate, the intensity of the workout and sweat rate are just a few variables that affect how much fluid you need. It is up to us to recognise the early warning signals of dehydration and the opposite, the rare, but often fatal, hyponatremia caused by too much water, and the detrimental effects that these can have, both on our bodies and on our performance.

Dehydration = *Fluid loss from under-drinking*

Hyponatremia = *Water-intoxication – low blood salt level due to abnormal fluid retention from drinking too much water*

You can always check that you are properly hydrated by inspecting the colour of your urine at the end of a workout – it should be light rather than dark, a pale straw-colour is ideal. Other symptoms, however, are quite similar to both dehydration and hyponatremia, so you need to watch out if you start to feel any of the following:

- Dizziness
- Headache
- Nausea
- Confusion and disorientation
- Muscle cramps
- Extreme fatigue

It is best to keep fluid levels topped up all day, not just during your workouts. A basic rule is that the heavier you are or the more intense the exercise, the more fluid you will lose. The British Dietetic Association guidelines state that the average person should drink 1½–2½ litres of fluid per day, which can be taken in all different drinks including water, milk, tea and coffee, and that this intake should be increased during hot weather or during and after physical activity.

A good method to assess how much fluid you personally need in addition to the daily guidelines is to weigh yourself immediately before and immediately after an intense workout and work out the amount of weight lost. An approximate calculation is that 1kg of weight corresponds to 1 litre of water; but because you also need to replace the ongoing losses of sweat during recovery, you should make up the loss with 1½ litres for every 1kg in weight loss. So if you are ½kg lighter at the end of a workout, you should be drinking ¾ litre of fluid in addition to what you may already have taken on board.

As you become accustomed to the amount of fluid you need, you can devise your drinking strategy so that you don't have to drink such large quantities in one fell swoop.

'In the first two hours of a race, use a more dilute solution of energy drink to overcome dehydration later in race. After two hours, use a thicker solution to overcome muscle glycogen depletion.' Andy Wadsworth, fitness consultant, personal trainer, mountain biker and world-class triathlete. Xterra Triathlon, World Champion.

Water alone is not enough

We know just from the taste of sweat that it is not made up of just water – it is salty, it makes your eyes sting and it can stain your clothes. Your sweat is actually made up of electrolytes, such as sodium, potassium, chloride and magnesium: minerals that are necessary for the body to function properly. Hyponatremia can occur on rare occasions during prolonged activities which involve heavy sweating. It is caused by drinking so much water that the sodium concentration in the blood becomes diluted to the extent that vital body functions are jeopardised. When you sweat, you lose approximately 2–3.4g of sodium per litre of sweat, and some people can actually lose as much as 1 litre of sweat per hour during a race. During long runs and endurance races, a sports drink with sodium and electrolytes, rather than simple water, will help prevent hyponatremia – try either a commercial isotonic drink or a home-made version (see recipes on page 46). When it is really hot, make sure that you keep up your salt intake with salty foods or salt tablets to minimise the risk of diluting your blood too much with pure water.

I have only ever had one experience of real dehydration. It was a truly horrific experience. My whole body went into 'shut-down' mode. Travelling in a little-known area on the coast of Colombia as a student, I had been sitting on a bus in the sweltering heat for many, many hours. We had recently flown in from London and I was acclimatised neither to the heat, nor the humidity. Towards the end of the journey I started to feel increasingly nauseous, weak and dizzy. It was only when I climbed down from the bus that I realised that my clothes were completely soaked through. You could actually wring them out. Too dizzy to walk, I could hardly even move. My very sensible boyfriend (later to become my husband!) bought me a litre of water which I immediately downed in one. I then continued to gulp down two further litres. However, it was only after a few mouthfuls of salty chicken broth an hour or so later that I started to feel slightly more alert. If the chicken's claw had not been protruding out of the bowl, I might have been able to stomach a little more!

'I felt sick for most of the day but ignored it and I ended up collapsing at the finish line on day five [of the Marathon des Sables] ... spent the last night of the race with a drip in my hand suffering from heat exhaustion. The temperature was over 40°C but I was shivering and freezing, then the vomiting started ...' Vicky Ryan, teacher, head of girls' games, marathon runner and member of the England mixed touch rugby. Completed the Marathon des Sables in 2006.

'Eat and drink before it is too late. Once, in a race, I crashed my bike and lost all my food and drink. By the time I got to the next feed station it was too late and no food or drink would get me back on track.' Llewellyn Holmes, personal trainer, triathlete and road/mountainbike racer. World Xterra Championships (British age group winner and 2nd place) and Ironman (3rd place).

'Water is boring and sports drinks are expensive and sickly.' This is a comment I hear all too frequently from my athlete friends, and it is true that some sweet commercial sports drinks, although effective, can get a bit much after a while. What's more, they can be quite expensive. The fact is that there are hundreds of hydrating foods that can really help your hydration strategy. Fruit, for instance, has a very high water content. What could be more refreshing than a sweet and succulent slice of watermelon, made up of 97 per cent water – high G.I. and perfect for straight after a workout? Fruit juices are also a great alternative for athletes, because they contain extra calories and vital minerals and vitamins. I tend to make a home-made sports drink out of blackcurrant juice diluted with water and a teaspoon of salt, or half apple juice and half water, also with salt (½ teaspoon of salt per litre is a good guideline). Dextrose tablets dissolved in water also work well.

Recipes For Homemade Isotonic Drinks

Recipe 1

Measure out 250ml pure unsweetened fruit juice (any flavour)
Add 250ml water to make a total volume of 500ml
Add a pinch of salt (about ⅕ teaspoon)
Mix together and stir or shake well. Chill in the fridge.

Recipe 2

Measure out 100ml squash (any flavour – full sugar)
Add 400ml water to make a total volume of 500ml
Add a pinch of salt (about ⅕ teaspoon)
Mix together and stir or shake well. Chill in the fridge.

'For obvious reasons, sticky energy drinks are not great as a self-spray cooling aid or to rinse sunglasses. So in future long events, I'll have two bottles: one filled with energy drink, the other with water.' Jean-Philippe Gervais, IT consultant, cyclist, triathlete and kayaker. Best event – Étape du Tour 2007

Fresh fruit, fruit juice or a smoothie straight after a run on a hot day make a delicious treat and will also help rehydrate you, especially if diluted with water, give you a little carbohydrate to replenish your glycogen stores and boost your vitamin and mineral levels.

Raw fruit and vegetables all have a high water content – melon, strawberries, apples, citrus fruits, red fruits, pineapple, kiwis, tomatoes, broccoli, carrots, peppers, spinach, cabbage, radishes ... the list is endless. Even some relatively dry foods contain a high percentage of water, such as beans, grains like couscous and rice, and pasta (foods which expand with water). In hot weather you can very easily base your everyday training diet on foods that include higher levels of water, while still providing your body with the correct level of carbohydrate, protein, vitamins and minerals.

Hot Go Faster hydration tips

- ***Drink before you are thirsty.*** *Drink regularly throughout the day and drink generously before your workout, during your workout and again immediately afterwards.*
- ***Replace lost fluid with a sports drink if you are exercising for over an hour.*** *Around 150–250ml sports drink with electrolytes and sodium every 20–30 minutes or so will keep up your energy levels and replace lost body salts. Practise during training so you know which you find palatable and your own tolerance for fluid in the stomach.*

- ***Make yourself drink at particular milestones when training,*** *for example, every two miles.*
- ***Snack on hydrating foods.*** *Keep a fruit salad in the fridge and buy a different selection of fruit every time you shop. Store packs of blueberries and forest fruits in the freezer to make delicious, hydrating smoothies.*
- ***Increase your salt intake in hot weather.*** *Remember that water alone will not replace nutrients lost through sweat. Eat savoury foods (marmite sandwiches after a run work wonders for me) and add a pinch of salt to your drink.*
- ***Schedule your workouts in hot weather.*** *Be careful about what time of day you train. Get out first thing in the morning, before the sun has had time to heat up the ground, or late in the evening when it has cooled down.*
- ***Acclimatise yourself.*** *If you are not accustomed to the heat, start cautiously and build up gradually. If you are planning to race in hot weather, try to get in some training in similar weather conditions beforehand and calculate your personal drinking strategy.*
- ***Wear appropriate clothing.*** *Wear loose-fitting clothes made from a high-tech material rather than cotton, which soaks up the sweat, clings to your skin and makes you even hotter. Wear a sweat-proof sunscreen and a hat.*
- ***Choose your route carefully in hot weather.*** *Choose shaded areas, tree-lined tracks or woodland trails, preferably where there is water, such as a drinking fountain, or run in small circuits so that you can stop to top up with water.*
- ***Don't just drink – pour water over yourself.*** *You can lose up to 70 per cent of your body heat through the top of your head, so pouring water over yourself really does cool you down. Use the showers provided in races.*
- ***Recognise the warning signals.*** *Don't exercise through heat cramps. Stop if you feel faint, weak, dizzy or confused – rest, get into the shade and drink a sports drink.*

Part Two

go faster recipes

introduction

If you are training for a specific event, your training schedule could last from anything between three to six months, working out five to six days a week. Fuelling your body can sometimes become literally that – fuelling up just like you might fill up your car with petrol. Resorting to your old faithful carbo meals to fill you up quickly can become tedious – how often can a person eat Spaghetti Bolognese, or whatever his or her favourite staple is, without getting ever so slightly bored with it? The recipes in this book will give you plenty of new ideas for tasty, mouth-watering and imaginative meals to maintain your energy levels and keep you healthy. They are intended to add a little nutritious and delicious zest to your training diet to help and inspire you to increase your repertoire of healthy, carb-rich, energy-boosting recipes.

Each recipe is accompanied by a breakdown of calories, protein, carbohydrate, fat, salt and fibre per serving. Please note that the serving sizes are generous on the whole; they are designed for the hungry athlete. The recipes are generally designed to serve 4, unless otherwise stated, so by all means cut back for fewer people or increase accordingly for more – these are healthy recipes suitable for an active family as well as those doing a specific training schedule.

Each recipe is also marked with an icon to indicate its suitability so that you can quickly and easily find which one is right for what you need:

Healthy meal for your general training diet

Good for endurance

Good for recovery

You will also find an approximate guideline of how long each recipe takes to prepare and cook. This should help you plan your meals around your busy training, work and/or family schedule. The majority of the recipes are very quick to prepare. There may be some ingredients with which you are less familiar but these can typically still be found in the supermarket rather than specialist delicatessens or health-food shops. Where this is not the case, I have suggested alternatives.

Important notes: oven temperatures are for a standard fan oven – you will need to add about another 20°C or 1–2 gas marks for a conventional oven. Also, unless stated, egg sizes are large and free-range; butter is unsalted; a glug of olive oil is approx. 1–2 tablespoons.

breakfast

'Breakfast is to be cherished – it is THE reason to get up in the morning. Why wait till you have punished yourself on a long ride to put fuel in the tank? Eat and be merry! Preferably a large, hot bowl of porridge. When you get home, it's lunchtime and you'll be a meal behind if you missed breakfast. And nutrition on the bike doesn't count as breakfast.' Michelle Lee, triathlete, marathoner, cyclist, duathlete, professional sportsperson, teacher, mum, sport and remedial massage therapist. World Duathlon 2006–08 (3rd); marathon personal best: 2:35.

'With a pre-training bowl of porridge, I felt I could keep going forever'. Adam Mason, TV sports rights manager, runner, cyclist, swimmer and skier. Best event – Étape du Tour 2007.

'My coach says that finishing 0.09 seconds away from a final place in the Nationals was down to my lack of breakfast – all I ate were two plain bagels, and I ended up swimming on empty.' Oliver Eyre, swimmer. Best event – National Swimming Championships 2007: 100m, 200m and 400m freestyle.

Go Faster Porridge, with Blueberries, Toasted Walnuts and Honey

The very best low-fat, low-G.I. endurance breakfast, whether you're running a marathon or doing an important presentation for work.

This is my fail-safe breakfast if I have got a big day ahead and you can guarantee that I will have this breakfast on the morning of a marathon. The oats have a very low G.I., meaning that the carbohydrate is released into your bloodstream slowly and therefore will sustain your energy levels and help prevent those 11 o'clock food cravings. What's more, studies show that a bowl of porridge can lower cholesterol. If I am running, I always make my porridge with water only as it is lighter on the stomach than milk. It is important that you use whole rolled porridge oats; they are less refined, more nutritious and they taste better – sweet and nutty. Pop the walnuts in the oven while you cook the porridge and you will be sitting down to breakfast within 10 minutes. Don't be put off by the fact that you have to wash up the saucepan afterwards, just pour cold water into the pan immediately after serving and the pan cleans really easily.

Nutrition per serving

Energy (kcal)	382	Protein (g)	12
Carbohydrate (g)	50	Fat (g)	15
Of which sugars (g)	19	Of which saturates (g)	2
Salt (g)	1.1	Fibre (g)	7

Serves 2
Cooking time – 10 minutes

100g whole rolled unrefined Scottish porridge oats
550ml water or milk, or half water and half milk
pinch of salt
150g fresh blueberries (or frozen blueberries, defrosted)
handful of walnuts
1 heaped tsp good-quality runny honey, or to taste (manuka is very good)

1. Preheat the oven to 160°C/gas mark 3.
2. Put the oats, water and/or milk into a pan with a pinch of salt. Bring to the boil over a high heat and then turn the heat down and simmer gently for about 5 minutes, stirring frequently. The porridge will become thick and creamy.
3. Meanwhile, pop the nuts onto a baking tray and roast in the oven for 5 minutes.
4. Pour the porridge into two warmed bowls, sprinkle with the blueberries and nuts and drizzle over the honey.

Homemade Fruit and Nut Muesli with Banana and Yoghurt

Great pre-exercise breakfast – tasty, sustaining and nutritious.

I am often quite disappointed with shop muesli. I don't seem to be able to find a combination that really suits my taste – there is either too much fruit, too little fruit, too many powdery oats or bits of dried banana, the one type of dried fruit I don't like! I know I am not alone in this quest for the perfect muesli; in fact, there is a whole 'muesli-holics' forum on the *Runner's World* website, on which people discuss their ideal muesli in great detail. Making your own muesli solves the predicament. It is also quite satisfying to know that you have all your favourite tasty goodies in the jar, so you don't have to pick out the bits you don't fancy. And you don't need to go to the health food shop for the ingredients; supermarkets stock a good variety of dried fruit and nuts nowadays.

Nutrition per serving

Energy (kcal)	600	Protein (g)	19
Carbohydrate (g)	90	Fat (g)	23
Of which sugars (g)	48	Of which saturates (g)	4
Salt (g)	0.3	Fibre (g)	8

Makes 2 good-sized portions
Prep time – 5 minutes

120g whole rolled unrefined Scottish porridge oats
30g raisins
15g crystallised ginger, chopped
25g soft dried pitted apricots (about 3), chopped
10g soft dried pitted dates (about 2), chopped
10g toasted hazelnuts, chopped
15g Brazil nuts, chopped into chunks
small handful of pumpkin seeds
small handful of sunflower seeds

1 banana
skimmed milk and low-fat natural yoghurt to serve

1. Mix the oats, fruit, ginger, nuts and seeds together. You can make a larger quantity of the dry ingredients and keep it in an airtight container if you like – it will keep for weeks.
2. To serve, pour the required amount into a bowl. Top with a chopped banana, some milk and a dollop of yoghurt. If you have a sweet tooth, you could drizzle some honey on top.

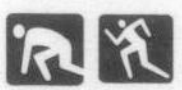

Birchermuesli

Good sustaining and nutritious breakfast for endurance – easy to eat, so good for before early morning sessions.

Birchermuesli was created by Dr Bircher-Benner in the 1890s for his patients in his Zurich hospital. It is an ideal healthy breakfast if you have a big day or a long training session ahead of you, but in fact the Swiss will eat Birchermuesli at other times, even as a light evening dish. Because you prepare it the night before all you have to do is remove the bowl from the fridge and eat it – it is even quicker than pouring out a bowl of cereal. What's more, the oats have been pre-soaked, so you can eat and digest this breakfast quickly. Birchermuesli will provide you with a good balance of nutrients – oats are of course *the* ideal slow-burning carbohydrate and, along with the fruit, they will give you fibre and help lower cholesterol; nuts are rich in omega-3 fatty acids, the milk and yoghurt provide some protein and on top of all this goodness you get vitamins from the fruit.

Nutrition per serving

Energy (kcal)	477	Protein (g)	15
Carbohydrate (g)	71	Fat (g)	13
Of which sugars (g)	45	Of which saturates (g)	2
Salt (g)	0.3	Fibre (g)	8

Serves 1
Prep time – 5 minutes

120g natural unsweetened muesli with fruit and nuts (or make your own – see Homemade Fruit and Nut Muesli, page 56)
skimmed milk to cover the muesli
splash of apple juice
good grating of nutmeg, or ¼ tsp ground cinnamon or cardamom
1 crisp, fresh apple, chopped or grated
natural yoghurt

runny honey to drizzle on top
small handful of almonds, lightly toasted

1. Pour over enough skimmed milk to cover the muesli generously and add a splash of apple juice. Mix in the nutmeg. You can use more apple juice and less milk if you prefer, it depends on your taste.
2. Leave for a couple of hours or overnight in the fridge.
3. Grate or chop an apple into the bowl before eating. Check the muesli is the consistency you like. You may need some more liquid to loosen it up. Add more fresh fruit, some toasted almonds or seeds for a bit of crunch, a dollop of yoghurt and some honey.

American Blueberry Pancakes

Good for recovery breakfast after Sunday morning exercise session.

I discovered American blueberry pancakes on my first visit to New York, when my husband ran the New York Marathon. Keen to get the full Big Apple experience, we got into the habit of having breakfast in a local 'all-American' diner. American pancakes are light and fluffy and are a great, fun way to get some high-G.I. carbs and protein into your body after some serious exercise. And of course you get a fantastic vitamin kick with the addition of the delicious blueberries, which are absolutely bursting with nutrients. I can't say that the lashings of maple syrup and the crispy bacon we ate on the side were quite so healthy, but when in Rome ... The art of cooking American pancakes is completely different to cooking our thin European-style pancakes. You need the flame down low and you need to let them cook through slowly. The Americans add sugar to their pancake mixture but I draw the line at this, on the basis that you then smother them in syrup.

Nutrition per serving

Energy (kcal)	303	Protein (g)	11
Carbohydrate (g)	47	Fat (g)	9
Of which sugars (g)	8	Of which saturates (g)	2
Salt (g)	2	Fibre (g)	3

Serves 4
Prep time – 5 minutes/Cooking time – 5 minutes

200g self-raising flour, sifted
2 tsp baking powder
¼ tsp freshly grated nutmeg
¼ tsp ground cinnamon
pinch of salt
1 whole egg plus 1 egg white

300ml buttermilk, or 150ml semi-skimmed milk mixed with 150ml low-fat natural yoghurt
2 tbsp melted butter or vegetable oil, plus a little more melted butter for frying
150g blueberries, fresh or frozen
extra blueberries and maple syrup to serve

1. Combine the flour, baking powder, nutmeg, cinnamon and salt in a bowl.
2. Whisk the egg white until it starts to form soft peaks.
3. Make a hole in the centre of the flour mixture, break the egg into it and then add the buttermilk or milk and yoghurt (or even just ordinary milk if you have no yoghurt).
4. Stir the wet ingredients quickly into the dry using a wooden spoon. Don't worry too much if it is not very smooth. Add the melted butter or oil and the blueberries and then fold in the egg white.
5. Brush the bottom of a frying pan with a little melted butter and then spoon in the pancake mixture. I like lots of fairly small pancakes, so I use a heaped tablespoon of mixture per pancake, but this is up to you.
6. After a few minutes you will see lots of air bubbles appear on the surface of the pancakes. This means it is time to flip them over. Cook them for a couple of minutes on the other side, and then serve them with extra blueberries on the side and maple syrup to pour over them, or just sprinkled with crunchy demerara sugar.

Breton Buckwheat Pancakes with Ham and Cheese

Good for a low-G.I. nutritious breakfast, brunch or even a light evening meal with a green salad. Will keep you sustained for hours.

Despite its name, buckwheat, or sarrasin, is a member of the rhubarb family and has absolutely nothing to do with wheat. It is naturally gluten-free and has a deliciously sweet, nutty flavour. It is traditionally used in Brittany in 'galettes de sarrasin', or buckwheat pancakes. Breton galettes can be filled with any number of fillings. You could try this recipe with traditional savoury fillings, such as slices of brie, goats' cheese, smoked salmon, caramelised onions or eggs, or with sweet fillings - bananas and syrup is one of my favourites. Buckwheat is a very good source of manganese, magnesium and dietary fibre. It contains flavonoids and good-quality protein, and is said to control blood sugar levels. It certainly keeps you full of energy for hours. The Bretons not only tend to make their galettes with dry Breton cider rather than milk and water, but they also wash them down with a few glasses of the delicious nectar. By all means try this, but not if you are about to go to the gym or run a half-marathon. This is my non-alcoholic breakfast version.

Nutrition per serving

Energy (kcal)	518	Protein (g)	24
Carbohydrate (g)	28	Fat (g)	35
Of which sugars (g)	2	Of which saturates (g)	21
Salt (g)	2.5	Fibre (g)	2

Serves 4 (makes 8–10 pancakes)
Prep time - 5 minutes/Cooking time - 5 minutes

For the pancakes

100g buckwheat flour

50g plain flour, wholemeal or white (the addition of plain wheat flour improves the texture of the galettes. If you want to make the pancakes gluten-free, just use 150g buckwheat flour instead)

pinch of salt
1 egg
100ml semi-skimmed milk
200ml water
30g melted butter plus extra butter to cook

For the filling
8–10 thin slices of good-quality cooked ham (1 per pancake)
200g grated cheese – Emmental, Gruyère or Cheddar

1. Mix the buckwheat and plain flour together, add a pinch of salt and make a small well in the centre for the egg.
2. Break the egg into the mixture and then add the milk and half the water.
3. Beat together with an electric hand whisk until the mixture is nice and smooth. Mix in the rest of the water and the melted butter. The mixture should be the consistency of thin cream.
4. If possible, leave the mixture to rest for a few hours or overnight.
5. Heat a pancake pan or large non-stick frying pan over a medium heat. Add a knob of butter and move the pan around so that the butter melts to cover the base of the pan. Lift the pan off the heat and add a small ladleful of the batter and quickly swirl it around so that you have a very thin layer of batter covering the whole of the pan. You can use a palette knife or an egg slice if you have one to spread out the mixture. Let this cook for 2 minutes over a medium heat, or until the pancake comes away easily from the pan when you shake it. Then toss the pancake over and cook for a minute or two on the other side.
6. Flip the pancake back over and then pop a very small knob of butter, a thin slice of ham and a tablespoon of grated cheese onto one half of the pancake.
7. Fold the plain half of the pancake over the filling and then fold in half again and cook on a very gentle heat for a minute or two until the cheese has melted.

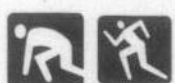

Date and Walnut Breakfast Muffins with Cinnamon Streusel

Low G.I., low fat, full of antioxidants, minerals and fibre, great for a wholesome and nutritious 'breakfast on the go' or as a pre-exercise energy boost before a lunchtime or evening workout.

These muffins are a wonderful excuse to eat cake for breakfast. They could be filled with any variety of fruit or dried fruit and nuts. The secret is to make them quickly and to avoid overmixing. If you do overmix, the muffin goes rather chewy and tough, so just fold the wet ingredients into the dry until they are just combined and then pop them into the oven. These muffins contain only a small amount of sugar as the dates add enough sweetness. By all means add a little extra sugar if you prefer a sweeter muffin with your morning cup of coffee. My kids like these muffins served warm with butter and honey as part of a Sunday brunch or after school.

Nutrition per serving

Energy (kcal)	286	Protein (g)	6
Carbohydrate (g)	35	Fat (g)	14
Of which sugars (g)	17	Of which saturates (g)	2.5
Salt (g)	0.4	Fibre (g)	2

Makes 12 muffins
Prep time – 5 minutes/Cooking time – 15–20 minutes

For the muffins

150g white self-raising flour
150g wholemeal self-raising flour
pinch of salt
2 tsp baking powder
1 tsp bicarbonate of soda
80g soft brown sugar
½ tsp ginger
½ tsp cinnamon
75g chopped walnuts

120g dates, chopped
2 eggs
90ml vegetable oil
1 tbsp runny honey
80ml semi-skimmed or skimmed milk
80ml low-fat natural yoghurt

For the cinnamon streusel topping
1 tbsp demerara sugar
1 tbsp plain flour
½ tsp cinnamon
25g butter, softened

1. Preheat the oven to 180°C/gas mark 4. Line a muffin tray with 12 muffin cases.
2. Make the cinnamon streusel topping: mix together the sugar, flour and cinnamon and then add the butter and rub in with your fingers until you have a crumbly mixture. Set aside to sprinkle on top before the muffins go in the oven.
3. Mix the white and wholemeal flour, salt, baking powder, bicarbonate of soda, sugar and spices together.
4. Add the walnuts and dates and combine.
5. Break the eggs into a separate bowl and add the oil, honey, milk and yoghurt.
6. Beat very lightly with a fork then pour the mixture into the bowl with the dry ingredients and combine quickly. The mixture will appear lumpy, but don't worry, just spoon it into the muffin cases, sprinkle the cinnamon streusel on top and pop into the oven for 15–20 minutes. They will rise and turn golden brown.
7. Cool on a wire rack and eat immediately.

Devilled Tomatoes on Toast

Nutritious low-G.I. breakfast, good for endurance, especially if you fancy a change from cereal or oats.

This is a really satisfying breakfast, and quick to prepare. The tomatoes and the wholemeal toast have a really low G.I. index and so will release energy to your bloodstream slowly and gradually. Tomatoes are brimming with nutrients, including vitamins C, A and B and minerals such as niacin, riboflavin, magnesium, phosphorous and calcium. They are also a good source of fibre and the antioxidant lycopene (good for fighting disease). You can play around with the ingredients to make the tomatoes as hot and spicy as you fancy, but this is how I like it.

Nutrition per serving

Energy (kcal)	190	Protein (g)	5
Carbohydrate (g)	22	Fat (g)	10
Of which sugars (g)	7	Of which saturates (g)	5.5
Salt (g)	2.5	Fibre (g)	3.5

Serves 2

Prep time – 5 minutes/Cooking time – 10 minutes

4 good-quality ripe tomatoes (for example on the vine), halved
20g softened butter
¼ tsp cayenne pepper
1 tbsp Worcestershire sauce
1 tsp cider vinegar
1 tsp English mustard
pinch of salt and black pepper
1 scant tsp sugar
2 slices good-quality wholemeal bread

1. Heat the grill to high.
2. In a bowl, mix together the butter, cayenne, Worcestershire sauce, vinegar, mustard and salt and pepper.

3. Put the tomatoes on a baking sheet, cut side up, and pop a knob of the butter mixture on each tomato half. Pour over any extra liquid that might not have been incorporated into the butter.
4. Sprinkle the sugar over the tomatoes.
5. Place under the grill for about 10 minutes until golden.
6. Meanwhile make your toast.
7. Place four tomato halves onto each slice of toast. Scrape any excess juices from the pan and pour over the tomatoes. Serve immediately.

Hot Oatcakes with Strawberries and Minted Maple Syrup

An excellent weekend brunch or a low-G.I., low-fat, hearty breakfast – good fuel for endurance.

These ultra-light little oatcakes make a delightful, quick, easy and balanced breakfast, containing protein, slow-burning carbohydrate, vitamins, calcium, great minerals and fibre. A fantastic start to the day if you plan to exercise or if you have a big day ahead of you. The mint in the maple syrup makes it slightly less sweet and is the perfect accompaniment to the strawberries. I sometimes warm the syrup and the strawberries together in a pan for a moment before pouring over the oatcakes.

Nutrition per serving

Energy (kcal)	187	Protein (g)	6
Carbohydrate (g)	30	Fat (g)	6
Of which sugars (g)	14	Of which saturates (g)	3
Salt (g)	0.6	Fibre (g)	3

Makes about 8 oatcakes
Prep time – 5 minutes/Cooking time – 5 minutes

2 tbsp fresh mint, very finely chopped
4 tbsp maple syrup
150g wholemeal self-raising flour
50g unrefined whole rolled porridge oats
½ tsp baking powder
½ tsp bicarbonate of soda
pinch of salt
15g caster sugar
2 eggs, lightly beaten
150ml milk
25g melted butter (optional)
40ml warm water
knob of butter for frying
400g strawberries

1. Mix together the mint and the maple syrup and leave for a few minutes to infuse.
2. Mix together the dry ingredients in a bowl and make a well for the eggs. Break the eggs into the well and then mix together quickly with a metal spoon, gradually adding the milk until you have a smooth batter.
3. Add the warm water and the melted butter. Don't let the mixture rest, use it immediately.
4. Heat a non-stick frying pan and melt a knob of butter in it.
5. Cook 3–4 oatcakes at a time over a gentle heat, using a scant tablespoon of batter for each cake – you do not want them too thick and they will rise anyway during the cooking process.
6. Cook for a minute or two until bubbles start to appear on top, then flip over and cook for 1 minute on the other side.
7. Serve immediately with the strawberries and the minted maple syrup.

Spiced Autumn Fruits Salad

Good for Sunday brunch or a quick, light breakfast. Also useful to store in the fridge for snacking.

This makes a really tasty breakfast served with Greek yoghurt and crunchy granola. The fruit compote is high in fibre, antioxidants and minerals, and eating it with yoghurt and granola gives you a balanced breakfast with protein, calcium, slow-burning carbohydrates and good fats from the nuts. I would top up this breakfast with a slice a wholemeal toast if I was planning an exercise session.

Nutrition per serving

Energy (kcal)	306	Protein (g)	3.5
Carbohydrate (g)	75	Fat (g)	1
Of which sugars (g)	74	Of which saturates (g)	0
Salt (g)	0.1	Fibre (g)	8

Serves 2

Prep time – 10 minutes/Cooking time – 15 minutes

1 large hard pear, cored and cut into wedges
1 good-quality sharp apple (such as Cox's), cored and cut into wedges
2 plums, halved and stoned
approx. 12 pieces of whole dried fruit – prunes, apricots or figs
2 cloves (optional)
1 cinnamon stick
2 star anise
1 bay leaf
zest of ½ an orange
1 tsp vanilla essence
1 tsp preserved ginger syrup (from a jar of stem ginger)
½–1 tbsp soft dark brown sugar
200ml apple juice
150ml water

1. Put all the ingredients except the apple into a saucepan and bring to a boil.
2. Simmer for about 10 minutes or until the dried fruit becomes plump and the fresh fruit is tender, but not too soft. Add the apple about 4 minutes before the end of cooking as it doesn't take as long to cook as the other fruit.
3. Spoon off the fruit into a bowl and boil the syrup at a high heat for 2 minutes, then leave it to cool before adding to the fruit. You can serve the compote warm or cold. It keeps well (and the flavours improve) for up to a week in the fridge.
4. Serve with Greek yoghurt and crunchy granola (see page 72).

Crunchy Granola

A tasty breakfast or snack to add a little variety to your training diet; packed with nutritious energy, slow-burning carbohydrates and good unsaturated fats from the nuts.

This granola is very versatile and really is so much better, and healthier, than the shop-bought version. It is delicious for breakfast with fresh fruit, fruit compote and yoghurt, or as a nutritious and tasty snack. One of my sons often has this granola when he returns hungry from school – he pours himself a small bowl and picks at it while he is doing his homework. Annette, a local running friend, sums it up in her comment on my gofasterfood blog: 'I've just made this granola and I know it's going to be a hit with my family. In fact, my husband just walked past and pinched some. He loved it!'

Nutrition per serving

Energy (kcal)	455	Protein (g)	10
Carbohydrate (g)	39	Fat (g)	29
Of which sugars (g)	16	Of which saturates (g)	3
Salt (g)	0.1	Fibre (g)	5

Makes about 6 servings
Prep time – a few minutes/Cooking time – 20 minutes

200g unrefined whole rolled porridge oats
250g mixed nuts and seeds (flaked almonds, sunflower and pumpkin seeds, walnuts, pistachios, pecans and hazelnuts)
½ tsp cinnamon
½ tsp ground ginger
2 tbsp honey or maple syrup
2 tbsp sunflower oil
2 tbsp water
100g mixed dried fruit (raisins, crystallised ginger, dried apricots, figs and/or dates), chopped (optional)

1. Preheat the oven to 180°C/gas mark 4.
2. Mix together the oats, nuts and seeds with the spices, honey, oil and water.
3. Spread the mixture evenly onto a large baking sheet.
4. Bake for 20 minutes until golden brown, turning the mixture after 10 minutes for it to brown evenly.
5. Leave to cool for 5 minutes or so. It will crisp up like magic.
6. Add the dried fruit if using.
7. Store in an airtight container for up to three weeks.

Smoked Salmon and Scrambled Eggs on Wholemeal Drop Scones

Good for a weekend brunch, post-exercise snack or light meal.

These little drop scones are as light as a feather and take moments to make. Nutritious and sustaining, this dish will provide a balance of protein, essential vitamins and minerals and cholesterol-reducing omega-3 fatty acids. Using wholemeal flour instead of refined white flour, they are a healthier version of the traditional drop scone, or scotch pancake, and are equally good with sweet or savoury accompaniments. Try them with smoked salmon and scrambled eggs for a special and nutritious weekend brunch treat.

Nutrition per serving

Energy (kcal)	477	Protein (g)	35
Carbohydrate (g)	45	Fat (g)	15
Of which sugars (g)	13	Of which saturates (g)	4
Salt (g)	5	Fibre (g)	4.5

Serves 2
Prep time – 5 minutes/Cooking time – 10 minutes

For the drop scones

100g wholemeal self-raising flour
1 tsp bicarbonate of soda
1 tbsp caster sugar
pinch of salt
1 egg
150ml semi-skimmed milk
knob of butter

For the smoked salmon and scrambled eggs

4 eggs
splash of milk
salt and plenty of black pepper
4 slices smoked salmon

knob of butter
lemon wedges, a few capers and chopped chives to serve

1. Prepare the scrambled egg ingredients first so you are ready to make them as soon as the scones are cooked. Lightly beat the eggs and the milk together with a pinch of salt and some black pepper.
2. To make the drop scones, mix together the dry ingredients in a bowl and make a well for the egg. Break the egg into the well and then mix together quickly with a wooden spoon. Gradually add the milk and continue mixing until you have a smooth batter.
3. Don't let the mixture rest, use it immediately.
4. Heat a non-stick frying pan and melt a knob of butter in it.
5. Drop a scant tablespoon of batter into the pan for each scone – depending on the size of your pan, you can probably cook about 6 at a time. A clever tip is to drop the batter from the tip of the spoon for round cakes and from the side of the spoon for oval cakes.
6. Cook gently for a minute or two until bubbles start to appear on the surface of the drop scones, then flip over and cook for 1 minute on the other side.
7. To cook the scrambled eggs, melt a knob of butter in a small saucepan and, when the butter starts to sizzle slightly, pour in the egg mixture. Cook on a low heat, stirring slowly until the mixture begins to thicken and starts to become creamy. Remove from the heat while still slightly runny and serve immediately – there is nothing worse than solid scrambled egg.
8. Allow up to about 4 scones per person – pile the scrambled egg and smoked salmon on top and sprinkle with chives and a good grind of black pepper. Scatter the capers around the side of the dish with a wedge of lemon to squeeze over the salmon.

soups and light meals

'Eat as much good food as possible whenever you can as you are burning so many calories.' Mavis Paterson a.k.a. Grannymave, 70, retired nurse, long-distance cyclist and runner. Best event – 4,500 mile transcontinental bike ride across Canada, 2008.

Butter Bean Soup with Crispy Pancetta

Nutritious pre-exercise lunch or light supper.

This is a really delicious, simple and extremely nutritious soup. Prepare it in advance and freeze it if you like, but quite frankly it only takes about 20 minutes to make. It tastes great with big cheesy croutons. Sometimes we have this for a Saturday lunch, after everyone has returned from their various morning activities: football, rugby, running, even orchestra. I leave out the pancetta and serve it up with bacon, lettuce and tomato sandwiches made with fresh bread straight out of the bread machine.

Nutrition per serving

Energy (kcal)	499	Protein (g)	23
Carbohydrate (g)	43	Fat (g)	27
Of which sugars (g)	10	Of which saturates (g)	11
Salt (g)	4	Fibre (g)	14

Serves 4
Prep time – 2 minutes/Cooking time – 20 minutes

30g unsalted butter
1 onion, peeled and chopped
1 clove garlic, peeled and crushed
2 bay leaves
3 x 400g tins of butter beans, drained and rinsed
1 litre good chicken stock
salt to taste
1 tsp sunflower oil for frying
extra virgin olive oil
8 rashers of pancetta or thin streaky bacon

1. Heat the butter in a pan and gently sweat the onion and garlic with the bay leaves in the butter for about 5 minutes until soft. Do not let the onion brown.
2. Add the butter beans and stir in for about 2 minutes.
3. Add the chicken stock, bring to the boil, cover and then simmer for about 15 minutes.
4. Take out the bay leaves and then whiz the rest in a liquidiser or with a hand-held blender until smooth and creamy. Taste and season with salt. I think pepper ruins the subtle flavour here, but you may need some more salt, depending on the saltiness of the stock you have used.
5. Heat a frying pan over a high heat and fry the bacon or pancetta in the oil until crisp. Drain on some kitchen paper to take away excess fat.
6. Warm the soup and serve in bowls, drizzled with a little extra virgin olive oil and topped with a couple of pieces of pancetta.

Dhal Soup with Coriander

Low-fat, low-G.I. midweek supper, high in cholesterol-lowering fibre, B vitamins, protein, iron and magnesium – extremely nutritious and perfect for vegetarians.

This soup is quite spicy with a lovely smooth texture and the occasional burst of coriander and cumin seeds. You may want to use just one chilli depending on your taste and the strength of the chillies you are using. You should find a good variety of lentils and pulses in the supermarket.

Nutrition per serving

Energy (kcal)	280	Protein (g)	19
Carbohydrate (g)	44	Fat (g)	4
Of which sugars (g)	2	Of which saturates (g)	0.5
Salt (g)	2	Fibre (g)	5

Serves 4
Prep time – 30 minutes soaking/Cooking time – 45 minutes

300g yellow lentils – a mixture of moong dhal, urad dhal and split peas is good
1½ litres fresh chicken stock or water
bunch of coriander leaves
1 tbsp oil
1 heaped tsp cumin seeds, or to taste
2 green chillies, chopped, with seeds remaining
2 cloves garlic, peeled and crushed
1 tsp turmeric
1 tsp salt
1 tsp garam masala
knob of butter
1 dried red chilli, crushed

1. Wash the lentils in hot water, soak for 30 minutes, then drain.
2. Add the water or stock to a pan and bring to the boil. Add the drained lentils and simmer for about 40 minutes on a low heat,

stirring occasionally. Remove any froth that forms on the top with a spoon.

3. Cool and the blend until smooth. Add the coriander and blend for another 10 seconds until the coriander is finely chopped.
4. Heat the oil in a non-stick pan and add the cumin seeds. When they start to sizzle, add the green chillies and the garlic and fry for 30 seconds.
5. Add the lentil mixture to the pan and then stir in the turmeric. Cook on a low heat for 5 minutes. (If the soup looks too thick, add some water).
6. Finally stir in the garam masala, season with salt (the amount will depend on the saltiness of your stock) and add a knob of butter.
7. Serve in bowls and sprinkle with the crushed dried chilli.

Chickpea, Sweet Potato and Spinach Soup

A good low-fat, low-G.I. carbohydrate option which works really well as a hearty lunch for hungry people on a cold or rainy day, especially if you are planning some sport later on, or as a quick and easy supper with some crusty granary bread. This soup is warming and spicy and is absolutely packed with goodness. Chickpeas are a great source of minerals and fibre and they provide a virtually fat-free source of protein, the fresh ginger is fantastic to use in your training diet as an anti-inflammatory and, of course, spinach is just brimming with nutrients including iron and other important minerals and vitamin C.

Nutrition per serving

Energy (kcal)	258	Protein (g)	10
Carbohydrate (g)	36	Fat (g)	9
Of which sugars (g)	10	Of which saturates (g)	1
Salt (g)	1.5	Fibre (g)	7

Serves 4
Prep time – 5 minutes/Cooking time – 20 minutes

2 tbsp olive oil
1 onion, peeled and finely sliced
2 sweet potatoes, or 1 large one, peeled and cut into small cubes
2 cloves garlic, crushed
2cm piece of root ginger, peeled and sliced very finely or grated
1 tsp cumin seeds, dry fried for one minute and crushed in pestle and mortar
½ tsp cinnamon
¼ tsp cayenne pepper
¼ tsp English mustard powder
1 x 400g can chickpeas
2 tomatoes, chopped or 100ml passata
1 tsp honey

1 litre vegetable or chicken stock
salt and freshly ground black pepper to taste
200g fresh spinach leaves

1. Heat the oil in a large saucepan and gently fry the onion for about 2 minutes.
2. Add the sweet potato, garlic and ginger and fry for a further minute or two. Add the cumin, cinnamon and cayenne and mustard powder and cook for 30 seconds, gently stirring the mixture all the time.
3. Stir in the chickpeas, the tomatoes and the honey and cook for 2 minutes, stirring frequently.
4. Stir in the stock and bring the mixture to the boil. Cover and simmer for 10 minutes until the sweet potato is tender.
5. Puree the soup in a blender until smooth. Season with plenty of salt and black pepper.
6. Pour back into the saucepan, stir in the spinach leaves and cook for a further minute or two until the spinach is wilted.
7. Serve in warmed soup bowls.

Roasted Parsnip Soup with Cumin and Chilli and Cheesy Croutons

Warming, high-G.I. soup – perfect for recovery after a morning workout.

This very warming and nutritious soup is even tastier because the parsnips are roasted first so they become sweet and caramelised. Parsnips contain a good amount of vitamin C, folate and potassium, but they do have a pretty high G.I. factor, especially when roasted. The carbohydrate in them will raise blood sugar levels rapidly, making this soup brilliant for recovery after a big workout on a cold winter morning. I serve the soup with cheesy croutons.

Nutrition per serving

Energy (kcal)	333	Protein (g)	8
Carbohydrate (g)	46	Fat (g)	14
Of which sugars (g)	15	Of which saturates (g)	4
Salt (g)	1.3	Fibre (g)	9

Serves 4
Prep time – 5 minutes/Cooking time – 35 minutes (+ 45 minutes to roast the parsnips)

For the soup

500g parsnips, roughly chopped
3 tbsp olive oil
1 ½ tsp cumin seeds
1 dried red chilli, crushed
salt and pepper
knob of butter
2 red onions, peeled and chopped
2 leeks, chopped
3 sticks of celery, chopped and with stringy bits removed
1–1 ½ litres water or chicken stock

For the cheesy croutons

12 slices of baguette
2 tbsp olive oil
50g grated cheddar cheese (optional)
4 tsp crème fraîche to serve (optional)

1. Preheat the oven to 190°C/gas mark 5.
2. Toss the parsnips in 2 tbsp of the olive oil and sprinkle with the cumin seeds, chilli, salt and pepper. Roast them on a baking tray in the oven for about 45 minutes until nicely caramelised.
3. Heat the remaining oil and a knob of butter in a large pan and sauté the onion very gently for 2 minutes. Add the leeks and celery, cover and continue to cook very gently for about 20 minutes until soft. Check that you do not let it burn by stirring occasionally.
4. Add 1 litre water or stock, parsnips (remember to scrape out all the cumin seeds left on the bottom of the baking tray and add them too) and a good sprinkle of salt and simmer for a further 10 minutes or so. Cool and then liquidise until smooth.
5. Check the consistency – the soup won't be nice if it is too thick, so add some more stock if you need to thin it out a little. Check for seasoning and serve warm with a dollop of crème fraîche and some cheesy croutons.
6. For the croutons, brush the slices of bread with some olive oil on both sides and cook in the oven for about 5 minutes or until crisp and golden, using the same baking tray that you cooked the parsnips in (so you get the leftover cumin flavours). Sprinkle the cheese on top halfway through the cooking if you like.

Fragrant Thai Hot and Sour Prawn Soup (Tom Yam Goong) with Noodles

Good for replenishing lost minerals and salts after a high-energy exercise session.

Tom Yam Goong is a wonderful chilli-hot soup which combines the sweet, sour, salty and hot characteristics of Thai cooking. I make a higher-carb 'endurance version' of this soup by adding rice or buckwheat noodles. The soup is refreshing, tastes exotic and is surprisingly easy to make. The prawns are an excellent source of protein and minerals such as selenium, iron, zinc and magnesium. You can add extra vegetables such as peppers or mangetout if you like.

Nutrition per serving

Energy (kcal)	335	Protein (g)	21
Carbohydrate (g)	51	Fat (g)	6
Of which sugars (g)	6	Of which saturates (g)	2
Salt (g)	3.5	Fibre (g)	3

Serves 4
Prep time – 10 minutes/Cooking time – 10 minutes

500g fresh raw, unpeeled prawns (or a pack of raw, peeled frozen prawns, defrosted)
1½ litres chicken stock
8 kaffir lime leaves
2cm piece of fresh ginger, peeled and sliced very finely
2 stalks lemon grass, outer layers removed, inner parts bashed with a rolling pin to release the flavour
150g mushrooms, finely sliced
2 tomatoes, chopped (optional)
6 spring onions, sliced diagonally
1 tsp chilli paste
3 red chillies, chopped finely, seeds removed if very hot
2 tbsp freshly squeezed lime juice

2 tsp palm sugar or brown sugar
2–3 tbsp Thai fish sauce
large bunch of fresh coriander leaves, roughly chopped
250g noodles (such as Thai rice noodles, soba or buckwheat noodles)

1. If using fresh, unpeeled prawns, peel the prawns, keeping the shells and heads, remove the dark vein and set the prawns aside. Place the shells and heads in a pan with the stock. Bring to the boil and simmer for 10 minutes.
2. Strain the stock through a sieve and discard the shells. If you are using peeled frozen prawns you will have to omit this stage.
3. Bring the stock to the boil again and add the lime leaves, ginger and lemon grass. Boil rapidly for 2 minutes and then turn down to a low heat.
4. Add the mushrooms, tomatoes, spring onions, chilli paste and chillies.
5. Add the prawns to the stock pan, then the lime juice, sugar and 2 tbsp fish sauce and simmer for a couple of minutes until the prawns turn pink. Taste and adjust the flavour with more chilli paste, fish sauce, sugar or lime juice if necessary.
6. Meanwhile, cook the noodles according to the pack instructions in a separate pan and drain.
7. Remove the lemon grass, as this is not nice to eat, then add the noodles.
8. Stir in the fresh coriander and serve in warmed bowls. You could serve some extra chillies on the side if you like a bit of extra heat.

Caribbean Root Vegetable Toss

Really tasty medium- to high-G.I. warm salad, good for recovery or for a rest day.

We tend to either roast root vegetables or put them into soups in this country, but in fact they can make a really tasty, colourful and satisfying salad. This salad is medium to high G.I. so I would normally make it as part of a recovery meal, perhaps for a rest day. Fennel seeds are generally available on the supermarket spice shelf and they are really worth keeping in your store cupboard as they can add a delicious and slightly alternative flavour to your cooking. I would generally serve this as a meal in itself with a hunk of crusty bread, or with a piece of grilled fish sprinkled with Cajun spices.

Nutrition per serving

Energy (kcal)	200	Protein (g)	5
Carbohydrate (g)	37	Fat (g)	4
Of which sugars (g)	25	Of which saturates (g)	1
Salt (g)	0.8	Fibre (g)	4

Serves 4
Prep time – 10 minutes/Cooking time – 15 minutes

1 sweet potato, peeled and sliced into 2cm wedges
½ small pumpkin, peeled and sliced into 2cm wedges (keep sweet potato and pumpkin pieces to a similar size)
2 tbsp cumin seeds
2 tbsp fennel seeds
200ml orange juice
2 firm bananas, peeled and sliced into 1cm chunks
2 red onions, peeled and sliced very finely
plenty of salt and black pepper
handful of fresh coriander leaves
2 spring onions, chopped
handful of chopped peanuts or cashew nuts, or toasted desiccated coconut to serve

1. Toast the fennel and cumin seeds in a dry pan, then crush together with a pestle and mortar
2. Steam the vegetables until just tender.
3. Heat up the orange juice in a pan, add the bananas, onions, vegetables, spices, salt and pepper and coriander leaves and arrange beautifully on a plate.
4. Serve warm, on a large dish, garnished with the spring onions and nuts.

Chicken Mango Wraps with Salsa and Rocket

A lovely fresh-tasting, healthy low-fat meal. Great for Saturday lunch if you have guests.

There is something very convivial about sitting at the table and assembling your own wrap. You put in exactly what you want, you eat it with your fingers (yes, you will definitely need napkins or kitchen towel with this meal), and there is always the temptation to pile on too much delicious spicy chicken and fresh salsa, which means you invariably end up with the whole thing falling apart on you. My children often request this dish for when they have friends over, and I don't mind this at all, as it is a really fun way of eating a whole variety of fruit and green vegetables, with the added benefit of good, low-fat protein from the chicken.

Nutrition per serving

Energy (kcal)	700	Protein (g)	36
Carbohydrate (g)	60	Fat (g)	38
Of which sugars (g)	43	Of which saturates (g)	10
Salt (g)	1.7	Fibre (g)	7

Serves 2

Prep time – 15 minutes + up to 24 hours for chicken to marinade/Cooking time – 10–15 minutes

For the chicken wraps

2 free range chicken breasts (leave skin on for extra flavour, or use skinless if you want to cut out the fat)
4 tortilla wraps
2 large handfuls of rocket or watercress
glug of balsamic vinegar
fresh coriander leaves to serve

For the marinade

2 tbsp mango chutney

½ tbsp madras curry paste
1 tsp ground coriander
1 tsp ground cumin
1 tbsp olive oil
1 tbsp lemon juice

For the yoghurt sauce
200ml low-fat natural yoghurt
pinch of chilli powder
½ tsp ground coriander
½ tsp ground cumin

For the salsa
1 mango, chopped into small cubes
6cm cucumber, chopped into small cubes
6 firm cherry tomatoes, chopped into small cubes
½ tsp coriander seeds, crushed in pestle and mortar
handful of fresh mint leaves, roughly chopped
handful of fresh coriander leaves, roughly chopped
juice of ½ a lime
2 tbsp olive oil

1. Mix the marinade ingredients together, add to the chicken and leave for at least 10 minutes, but up to 24 hours in the fridge if you can.
2. Heat the grill to high. Place the chicken on a strong piece of aluminium foil, folded up at the sides around the chicken to catch the juices.
3. Cook the chicken under the grill for about 10–15 minutes, coating frequently with the marinade, including the lumps of mango from the chutney. Turn the chicken halfway through cooking. When the chicken is almost cooked, turn it skin side up so that it can crisp up.
4. Meanwhile prepare the yoghurt sauce. Mix together the yoghurt, chilli powder, ground coriander and cumin and chill until the chicken is ready to serve.

5. To make the salsa, mix all the salsa ingredients in a bowl. You can use green, red or yellow peppers as well if you like.
6. Put the rocket into a serving bowl.
7. Wrap the tortilla wraps in foil and warm them in the oven for a few minutes.
8. Carve the chicken breasts into diagonal strips, and place on a serving dish. Discard any fat in the foil tray and then add a glug of balsamic vinegar and scrape off the tasty bits stuck on the foil. Pour over the chicken. Decorate with coriander leaves.
9 Arrange the salsa, yoghurt sauce, chicken and rocket in separate dishes on the table and then prepare your wraps. Add a little bit of everything to your tortilla, roll it like a pancake, cut it in half, pick it up and eat it.

Green Mango Salad

This salad takes no time to prepare and is fresh, healthy and full of flavour.

Green, unripe mangoes have a firmer flesh and are not as sweet as the ripened ones we are used to eating as a fruit here in the UK. You can buy them in oriental food stores and they are sometimes even available in the local supermarket. Use any mango as an alternative, but it needs to be still firm. Mangoes are one of those fruits that seem to have everything – they're rich in dietary fibre and carbohydrate, and also contain vitamins A, C and E, B vitamins, potassium, copper and amino acids. A pain to peel and very messy to eat, but definitely worth the effort. Don't worry too much about exact quantities, just throw it all together. If you want to make this salad more substantial, you could mix in some prawns or thin slices of roast duck or serve it with a fresh tuna steak.

Nutrition per serving

Energy (kcal)	232	Protein (g)	6
Carbohydrate (g)	42	Fat (g)	5
Of which sugars (g)	30	Of which saturates (g)	1
Salt (g)	2.8	Fibre (g)	7

Serves 4 as a starter, 2 for a main course
Prep time – 10 minutes

2 green mangoes – if you cannot find these, use another type of mango but ensure that it is unripe
1 tbsp lime juice
1 tsp Thai shrimp paste
1 tbsp finely ground roasted peanuts (you can use peanut butter or satay sauce for the sake of speed)
2 tbsp Thai fish sauce
1 tbsp palm sugar or soft brown sugar
1 tbsp chilli paste
a little finely chopped fresh ginger

bunch of fresh mint leaves or Thai basil, chopped
bunch of coriander leaves, chopped
1 small fresh green chilli, chopped finely
2 spring onions, finely chopped
crisp green salad leaves (Romaine or Cos for instance) and chopped peanuts to serve

1. Peel and core the mangoes and slice very finely into thin shreds with a peeler or a mandolin, or even grate with a grater.
2. Gently combine all the ingredients and taste to see if you need a little more sugar, lime juice, fish sauce or chilli to balance the flavours.
3. Serve on the salad leaves and sprinkle with chopped peanuts.

Pork Tenderloin and Chorizo Kebabs with a Salad of Lamb's Lettuce, Sauteed Apple and Bacon

Rich in protein, vitamins and minerals - a bit of indulgence if you fancy a break from carbs. Great recipe for an informal supper party or barbecue.

Lamb's lettuce has tender, dark, oval leaves and a lovely tangy flavour. It is also rich in vitamins A and C, iron and folic acid. If you can't get hold of it, use spinach or watercress instead. Although I absolutely love pork, I try not to eat it too often, as it is pretty high in cholesterol. The same goes for chorizo, but it is used sparingly in this recipe and it does make for the most delicious kebabs. Try to buy the chorizo in its whole 'sausage' form rather than sliced - it is usually in a pack on the shelf with other prepacked whole salamis in the supermarket. When you thread the kebabs, make sure the bread is next to the chorizo so that the juices run into it - it is really mouthwatering. If you can't find sage then use tarragon instead.

Nutrition per serving

Energy (kcal)	650	Protein (g)	38
Carbohydrate (g)	26	Fat (g)	44
Of which sugars (g)	8	Of which saturates (g)	6
Salt (g)	4.3	Fibre (g)	4

Serves 4

Prep time - 10 minutes/Cooking time - 10–15 minutes plus a few minutes for the salad

You will need 8 skewers

For the kebabs

2 x 175–200g tenderloins of pork, fat removed, cut into 12 x 2.5cm cubes

24 sage leaves

24 x 2cm cubes bread (granary best)

2 green peppers
1 chorizo sausage cut into 12 x 2cm pieces

For the marinade
6 tbsp olive oil
juice of 1 lemon
12 sage leaves, chopped
1 tsp paprika
salt and pepper

For the salad
2 large handfuls (or a small bag) of lamb's lettuce, spinach or watercress
1 apple, cored and chopped into small chunks
100g smoked bacon pieces or pancetta, chopped into small cubes
knob of butter
olive oil
white balsamic or white wine vinegar

1. If you are using bamboo skewers, soak them into a bowl of water for ½ hour or so before using – otherwise they will burn.
2. In a bowl, mix the olive oil, lemon juice, chopped sage and paprika with a pinch of salt and a few grinds of black pepper. Add the kebab ingredients and make sure everything is well coated. Leave until the kebab skewers are ready.
3. Thread the kebabs – this order is best: green pepper, pork, sage leaf, bread, chorizo, green pepper etc.
4. Cook the kebabs under a medium to hot grill or on the barbecue for about 10 minutes, turning so that all the sides get cooked. The bread should go crispy and the pork should be just cooked through.
5. To make the salad, sauté the bacon until crisp in a good knob of butter and a little olive oil. Add the apples and cook until just on the verge of going soft.
6. Add salt and plenty of black pepper, plus a little vinegar.
7. Add to the lettuce just before serving, scraping all the juices off the pan.

Salad of Figs, Parma Ham, Rocket and Nasturtium Flowers with a Honey Balsamic Dressing

If you are in training, you may want to serve this as a starter or as an accompaniment to a copious bowl of butter bean or chickpea soup.

This is a really special salad. It won't give you much endurance, but it is full of flavour, vitamins and protein and a joy to eat. I often make it for lunch or a light supper when there are figs in the shops and when the garden is overrun with nasturtiums. The nasturtiums are not absolutely necessary; although they do look pretty and taste fantastic, they are only in the shops every now and then. They have a strong peppery flavour so if you use rocket or watercress you can get a certain amount of pepperyness without them. This salad is good with goats' cheese – cut some rounds of goats' cheese and melt them on some croutons of bread.

Nutrition per serving

Energy (kcal)	335	Protein (g)	12
Carbohydrate (g)	45	Fat (g)	13
Of which sugars (g)	24	Of which saturates (g)	5
Salt (g)	2.6	Fibre (g)	4

Serves 4
Prep time – 10 mins

For the salad

4 large handfuls of rocket leaves
4 ripe fresh figs
6–8 nasturtium flowers
4 slices Parma ham
12 slices French bread
12 rounds soft goats' cheese

For the dressing

2 tbsp olive oil

1 dessertspoon white balsamic vinegar

1 dessertspoon honey

salt and pepper

1. Mix the dressing ingredients together.
2. Toast the bread. Place a round of cheese onto each slice and grill until golden.
3. Arrange the salad ingredients on 4 plates and pour over the dressing.
4. Serve immediately.

Carpaccio of Vegetables with Sesame

Refreshing and hydrating salad, great as a starter or a light lunch with some pitta bread and falafel.

This is a vegetable version of the traditional carpaccio, a dish of beef or tuna sliced incredibly thinly and served raw. I first made this salad for lunch whilst on holiday in France. We had set out far too late for our early morning run (something that happens all too often when you are trying to squeeze training into a family holiday) and by the time we returned it was lunchtime and we were dying of thirst. This salad seemed to satisfy our hunger and quench our thirst brilliantly, and it was very fresh and flavoursome.

Nutrition per serving

Energy (kcal)	150	Protein (g)	4
Carbohydrate (g)	9	Fat (g)	11
Of which sugars (g)	8	Of which saturates (g)	1.5
Salt (g)	0.6	Fibre (g)	4

Serves 4
Prep time – 15–20 mins

2–3 firm tomatoes, sliced thinly into rounds
1 yellow pepper
1 green pepper
handful of mushrooms
1 cucumber
1 bulb of fennel
juice of ½ a lemon
2 tbsp extra virgin olive oil
1 tbsp sesame oil
1 tbsp toasted sesame seeds
1 tsp cumin seeds, dry roasted and crushed in a pestle and mortar
salt and freshly ground black pepper
large bunch of mixed fresh herbs (flat-leaf parsley, mint, coriander)

1. Make sure the vegetables are chilled. Cut the vegetables as thinly as you possibly can, using a mandolin if you have one or a really sharp knife. The cucumber should be cut into long strips, like large ribbons. Put all the vegetables apart from the tomatoes into a large bowl.
2. Mix together the lemon juice, olive oil and sesame oil, the cumin seeds, sesame seeds, ¾ of the herbs and the salt and pepper and pour over the vegetables, keeping a little back to drizzle over the tomatoes. Mix gently with your hands.
3. Arrange the tomatoes around the outside of a large plate and then pile the rest of the vegetables into the middle of the plate. Drizzle the rest of the dressing over the tomatoes.
4. Sprinkle with sesame seeds and the rest of the fresh herbs.

Frisée Salad with Oven-roasted Walnuts, Parma Ham, Tomatoes and Mozzarella

A good starter or light lunch; low carb but packed with nutrition.

An ideal, simple and delicious midweek treat, this salad is packed with flavour and nutrition and is substantial enough for a main meal. Walnuts are a great superfood, high in omega-3 fatty acids and antioxidants; the tomatoes are a rich source of vitamins and antioxidants and, of course, the Parma ham and mozzarella add both flavour and protein. You will really notice the difference if you focus on quality ingredients for this salad – buffalo mozzarella has a wonderful flavour if you can get it, but if not regular mozzarella will work just as well. Mop up the juices with some crusty fresh multi-grain bread.

Nutrition per serving

Energy (kcal)	595	Protein (g)	23
Carbohydrate (g)	37	Fat (g)	40
Of which sugars (g)	9	Of which saturates (g)	11
Salt (g)	4.5	Fibre (g)	5

Serves 2
Prep time – 5 mins/Cooking time – 10 mins

For the salad

4 slices Parma ham
6 slices French baguette or ciabatta (optional)
1 tbsp olive oil
large handful of walnuts
1 frisée lettuce
2–3 medium vine tomatoes
1 buffalo mozzarella
handful of flat-leaf parsley

For the dressing

1 tsp Dijon mustard
½ tbsp good-quality balsamic vinegar

squeeze of lemon juice
2 tbsp fruity olive oil
small clove garlic, crushed
salt and pepper

1. Preheat the oven to 180°C/gas mark 4.
2. Mix up the dressing in a nice big salad bowl. Leave the salad servers crossed over in the bowl (this creates a gap between the salad and the dressing and stops it going soggy). Alternatively, mix the dressing in a separate bowl and keep to one side.
3. Arrange the Parma ham and the baguette slices (if using) on a baking tray, drizzle each side with olive oil and cook in the oven for 8–10 minutes until the bread is golden and the ham is crispy.
4. Bake the walnuts on a separate baking tray for 5 minutes (keep an eye on them as they can burn very quickly).
5. Meanwhile, wash the lettuce and remove any tough outer leaves. Shake off the excess water and pull the leaves apart with your fingers. Pile into the salad bowl on top of the salad servers.
6. Slice the tomatoes and arrange them on top of the lettuce. Break the mozzarella into rough lumps and add to the salad.
7. Top with the walnuts, Parma ham, the parsley and the croutons.
8. Serve straight away, mixing in the dressing at the last moment.

Oven-roasted Peppers

A colourful, nutritious and warming dish to add variety and colour to your diet.

I first discovered this classic recipe as a 17 year old when, working as an au pair in Germany, I was sent out to buy 'a kilo of paprika'. Much to my employer's dismay, I returned with an enormous bag of ground paprika, unaware that the German word for 'red pepper' was indeed 'Paprika'! Brightly coloured peppers are rich sources of vitamin C and vitamin A (the antioxidant beta-carotene) and also contain good amounts of fibre and minerals such as potassium. These peppers caramelise in the oven and make a delicious starter or light lunch. Sometimes we eat them with spicy chickpea cous-cous if we need to increase our carbohydrate intake.

Nutrition per serving

Energy (kcal)	177	Protein (g)	7
Carbohydrate (g)	11	Fat (g)	12
Of which sugars (g)	9	Of which saturates (g)	4
Salt (g)	1.3	Fibre (g)	4

Serves 4
Prep time – 5–10 minutes/Cooking time – 20 minutes

4 red peppers, or a mixture of yellow, orange and red peppers, cut in half lengthways, with seeds removed
4 medium tomatoes, sliced quite thinly (or some sugocasa, if you have no fresh tomatoes)
2 cloves garlic, crushed
4–6 tinned anchovies, chopped finely
handful of fresh basil leaves, chopped, keep some back to sprinkle on top
plenty of freshly ground black pepper (no salt needed because of the anchovies)
2 tbsp extra virgin olive oil
1 tbsp good-quality balsamic vinegar
50g feta cheese (optional)

1. Preheat the oven to 220°C/gas mark 7.
2. Place the pepper halves on to a baking tray so that they fit snugly. Into each pepper half, place even amounts of the tomato, garlic, basil and anchovies.
3. Drizzle the olive oil over the peppers and season with some black pepper, then place into your really hot oven.
4. Roast for about 20 minutes, or until soft and caramelised (they should be going a little black around the edges to be at their best).
5. Take out of the oven, sprinkle over some fresh basil leaves, some more black pepper and the balsamic vinegar (you could also add some feta cheese here) and eat, soaking up the juices with some chunks of crusty bread.

Vegetable Tian

A healthy, balanced, light supper.

An authentic French tian is served in a terracotta dish of the same name and is basically layered vegetables cooked in the oven, a little like a gratin. It is a great way of eating vegetables and can be a meal in itself or served as an accompaniment to meat or fish. I love it with something simple like grilled lamb chops and plain couscous. The majority of the vegetables in this recipe are low G.I. and the celeriac is an excellent source of potassium and vitamin C, but you can use whatever vegetables you have available as long as you include the garlic, onions or leeks and a root vegetable like potatoes and celeriac. You could save time by slicing the firmer vegetables – the potatoes, celeriac, aubergine and courgettes in a food processor if you have one. I make it without the potatoes if I am serving it with couscous.

Nutrition per serving

Energy (kcal)	340	Protein (g)	15
Carbohydrate (g)	36	Fat (g)	16
Of which sugars (g)	18	Of which saturates (g)	6
Salt (g)	1	Fibre (g)	10

Serves 4 as a main course or 6–8 as a vegetable accompaniment

Prep time – 15 minutes/Cooking time – 50 minutes

You will need 1 gratin dish, about 34cm x 24cm

2 tbsp good olive oil, plus a little for cooking the leeks
2 leeks or 1 large onion, sliced thinly
3 courgettes, sliced thinly lengthways
2 red peppers and 3 long green peppers, cut into quarters lengthways (so they can lie as flat as possible)
1 large aubergine, sliced thinly lengthways
1 celeriac root, sliced thinly
4 tomatoes, sliced thinly
4 potatoes, peeled and sliced thinly

2 cloves garlic, peeled and crushed, plus 1 extra clove, peeled, for rubbing the dish with
large handful of fresh thyme or basil leaves (or use 1 tbsp pesto if you have a jar in the fridge)
salt and pepper
100g Gruyère cheese (optional), grated

1. Preheat the oven on to 180°C/gas mark 4. Rub the gratin dish all over with a clove of garlic and brush with a little oil.
2. Gently sauté the leeks until soft.
3. Build up the tian by arranging the vegetables in layers so that they fit tightly together. Layer each vegetable in turn. After each layer of vegetable, scatter over a few herbs, some garlic, some salt and pepper and a drizzle of olive oil.
4. When you have completed all the layers, cover the dish tightly with foil and pop it in the oven for about 30 minutes.
5. After 30 minutes, remove the foil and sprinkle over the cheese if you are using it. Bake for a further 20 minutes until the top is golden and the vegetables are tender. You can test that the potatoes are cooked with a fork or a skewer.

pasta

'We ate spaghetti in Little Italy – is there any better way to spend the night before a marathon?' Mark Collingwood, solicitor and marathon runner (personal best: 3:24). Best event – Amsterdam Marathon 2006.

'My favourite meal the night before an event is something simple like pasta. Don't overeat as your body can only store so much glycogen. It is easy to get gluttony and carbo-loading a little confused – well, it is for me anyway.' Adam Bardsley, Managing Director, Ironman (personal best: 10:28) and marathon (personal best: 2:41) runner. Best event – Ironman France 2008.

'In the prairies there were no shops and we were camping, so spaghetti and a can of chilli sauce was as good as it got.' Mavis Paterson a.k.a. Grannymave, 70, retired nurse, long-distance cyclist and runner. Best event – 4,500 mile transcontinental bike ride across Canada, 2008.

'The old clichéd pasta the night before works for me as long as it's not too late!' Vicky Ryan, teacher, head of girls' games, marathon runner and member of the England mixed touch rugby. Completed the Marathon des Sables, 2006.

Conchiglioni with Roasted Tomato Sauce

Excellent balanced, healthy low-fat, quick-fix meal for training and endurance and great for pre-race carbo-loading.

Conchiglioni are basically enormous pasta shells – you can find them on the pasta shelf of most supermarkets. The conchiglioni and the tomatoes have a low G.I., making the dish ideal for the night before a big workout. In fact, this is one of my favourite pre-race meals as it is so light on the stomach. The tomatoes are rich in vitamin C, vitamin A and B vitamins (niacin and riboflavin), magnesium, phosphorous and calcium, and are also a good source of fibre and the antioxidant lycopene (good for fighting disease). The cheese adds a little protein to the dish. I like to slow roast tomatoes because it gives them a lovely intense flavour.

Nutrition per serving

Energy (kcal)	639	Protein (g)	22
Carbohydrate (g)	100	Fat (g)	19
Of which sugars (g)	12	Of which saturates (g)	6
Salt (g)	1.8	Fibre (g)	6

Serves 4

Prep time – 2 minutes/Cooking time – 1 hour, but you only have to stir every now and then

8 decent-sized vine tomatoes
1 tbsp balsamic vinegar
2 tbsp olive oil
1 tsp demerara sugar
plenty of salt and black pepper
2 cloves of garlic, peeled and crushed
½ bottle sugocasa (like passata, but not so smooth; you can use 4 more fresh chopped tomatoes instead if you have them, or a small tin of chopped tomatoes)
1 small dried chilli, flaked (optional)
bunch of fresh basil, chopped, saving a few leaves whole for decoration

4 rashers streaky bacon or prosciutto (optional)
500g Conchiglioni pasta shells
1 tsp olive oil to drizzle over pasta
100g feta cheese, cubed

1. Preheat the oven to 170°C/gas mark 3.
2. Cut the tomatoes in half and place cut side up on a low-sided baking tray. Sprinkle over the balsamic vinegar, olive oil, sugar, salt and pepper and cook for 30–40 minutes until the tomatoes are soft and starting to caramelise.
3. Add the garlic after 30 minutes or about 5 minutes before you remove the tomatoes from the oven.
4. Transfer to a saucepan, scraping off all the caramelised bits as well, add the sugocasa and chilli if you are using it, and cook very gently, covered, for another 20 minutes or so, stirring every now and then.
5. Taste and add more balsamic, olive oil and seasoning if you think it needs it. Add the chopped basil at the last minute.
6. Grill the bacon until really crispy.
7. Cook the pasta shells in salted water according to pack instructions – warning, you need a big saucepan. Drain the pasta, reserving some of the cooking liquid to stop it getting sticky, and drizzle over some olive oil.
8. Serve the pasta in large individual pasta dishes with some sauce on top. Place a slice of bacon on top with some basil leaves and pieces of feta sprinkled over.

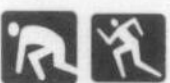

Fusilli Bucati Lungui alla Puttanesca

Healthy, low-G.I., low-fat dish, packed with nutrients.

This is a gutsy dish, quite spicy, very satisfying and great as a meal the night before a race or as part of your training schedule. Fusilli bucati lungui are available in most supermarkets and are tightly wound spirals of pasta, a little thicker than spaghetti, with a hole running through the middle of the strand. They are good fun to eat and go really well with this pungent puttanesca sauce. This is one of those 'store cupboard' pasta dishes that you can make when you haven't been able to get to the shops – as long as you have the basic ingredients of olives, anchovies, capers, chilli and garlic (things like the cherry toms and fresh herbs are nice to have but not essential), you can rustle up this dish with spaghetti, spaghettini, rigatoni, penne or whatever pasta comes to hand. It is surprisingly healthy, with omega-3 from the anchovies and vitamin C from the herbs and the garlic. Tomatoes in any form are full of nutrients and there is a good portion of low-G.I. carbohydrate from the pasta. A word of warning – wash your hands after you have crushed the chillies. I once forgot to and then took out my contact lenses later in the day – a painful experience.

Nutrition per serving

Energy (kcal)	682	Protein (g)	24
Carbohydrate (g)	104	Fat (g)	22
Of which sugars (g)	15	Of which saturates (g)	3.5
Salt (g)	2	Fibre (g)	7.5

Serves 4
Prep time – 5 minutes/Cooking time – 15 minutes

500g fusilli bucati lungui
2 tbsp olive oil
4 cloves of garlic, peeled and very finely sliced
2 whole dried chillies, crushed
50g tinned anchovies, drained and chopped roughly

2 tbsp capers, rinsed
handful of pitted black olives, chopped roughly
10 sun-dried tomatoes
1 x 400g tin of chopped tomatoes
200g cherry tomatoes, halved
2 tbsp fresh flat-leaf parsley, chopped
2 tbsp fresh basil leaves, chopped, plus some extra leaves for decoration
freshly ground black pepper
splash of balsamic vinegar
2 tbsp extra virgin olive oil
fresh parmesan shavings

1. Heat 2 tbsp oil in a medium saucepan and gently fry the garlic for a minute. Then add a dried chilli and the anchovies. Cook gently for a few minutes and then add the capers, the olives and the sun-dried tomatoes.
2. Add the can of tomatoes and cook, covered, for about 10 minutes, then add the cherry tomatoes and cook for a further 2 minutes or so until the tomatoes become a little soft. Finally, add the herbs, plenty of freshly ground black pepper and a splash of balsamic vinegar. Check for seasoning – you may need the other chilli but you probably will not need any salt because of the anchovies and the capers.
3. Meanwhile, bring a large saucepan of salted water to the boil and cook the fusilli according to the instructions on the pack. When the pasta is al dente, drain it and add it to the sauce. Add the extra virgin olive oil, stir it all together and then serve it up. Decorate with some torn up basil leaves and shavings of parmesan cheese.

Wholewheat Fettuccine with Jambon de Bayonne and Creamy Hazelnut Sauce

A balanced, low-G.I. carbohydrate dish, good for endurance and highly nutritious.

This is just delicious. Hazelnuts have a fantastic flavour, especially when they are lightly roasted. They are also really nutritious, high in antioxidants and an excellent source of vitamin E, dietary fibre, magnesium and heart-healthy B vitamins. If you cannot find Jambon de Bayonne, then any type of cured ham such as Serrano or Parma ham will be fine.

Nutrition per serving

Energy (kcal)	617	Protein (g)	27
Carbohydrate (g)	87	Fat (g)	20
Of which sugars (g)	6	Of which saturates (g)	5
Salt (g)	1.5	Fibre (g)	5

Serves 4

Prep time – 10 minutes/Cooking time – 10 minutes (you can prep the sauce while the pasta is cooking)

50g whole hazelnuts
450g fettuccine
pinch of salt
200g ricotta cheese
¼ tsp nutmeg, grated
1 clove of garlic, peeled and crushed
1 tbsp olive oil
1 leek, finely sliced
4 slices of Jambon de Bayonne, torn into shreds
freshly ground black pepper
a few fresh basil leaves

1. Preheat the oven to 180°C/gas mark 4.
2. Pop the hazelnuts on a baking tray and bake in the oven for about 5 minutes until lightly toasted.

3. Bring a large saucepan of salted water to the boil and cook the fettuccini according to pack instructions.
4. Meanwhile, blitz the hazelnuts, a pinch of salt, the ricotta, a good grating of nutmeg and the garlic in a blender until you have a smooth paste.
5. Heat the olive oil in a large frying pan, add a tbsp of water and very gently sauté the leek until it is soft and translucent.
6. Drain the pasta when it is cooked, reserving just a small ladleful of the cooking water. Add the pasta to the pan with the leeks, stir in the hazelnut sauce and add the ham.
7. Serve immediately with freshly ground pepper and the basil leaves. This pasta tastes very good with a fresh tomato salad.

Spaghetti with Toasted Pine Nuts, Fresh Basil and Parmesan Topped with Crispy Pancetta

Top of my list as the perfect dish for the night before a marathon. In those few days preceding a marathon, when it is all about loading up on carbs, you really do not want to be fussed with complicated dishes, and this dish is simple, quick, tasty, packed with good calories, the right balance of carbs, protein and fat and yet not too heavy. In fact, this meal tends to settle my nerves and I always seem to sleep well after it. I tend to limit the amount of fibre I eat the night before a race as I had a bad experience during the New York Marathon a few years ago which involved rather too many Portaloo stops, so I use regular spaghetti, but you can also use the wholewheat version if you like.

Nutrition per serving

Energy (kcal)	833	Protein (g)	27
Carbohydrate (g)	86	Fat (g)	45
Of which sugars (g)	5	Of which saturates (g)	10
Salt (g)	2.7	Fibre (g)	6.5

Serves 4
Prep time – a few minutes to heat up the pasta water/ Cooking time – 10–15 minutes

50g pine nuts
450g spaghetti
8 slices pancetta or streaky bacon
200g good-quality pesto
2 handfuls of fresh basil leaves, roughly torn, plus a few whole leaves to serve
freshly ground black pepper
plenty of parmesan cheese, shaved

1. Preheat the oven to 180°C/gas mark 4.
2. Gently roast the pine nuts in the oven for about 5 minutes until golden – keep checking them as they are easy to burn.
3. Bring a large pan of salted water to the boil and cook the spaghetti according to pack instructions until al dente.
4. Meanwhile, grill the bacon until crispy. Pour the pesto into a small saucepan and warm over a gentle heat.
5. Drain the spaghetti and pop it back in the pan with a good ladleful of the cooking water to stop it sticking.
6. Add the pesto and the torn basil leaves, the pine nuts, plenty of black pepper and as much parmesan as you want. Toss the spaghetti and serve in a big bowl in the centre of the table with the crispy pancetta and extra basil leaves on top for decoration.

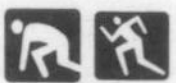

Spaghetti with Spinach and Pancetta

A simple and balanced carbo-loading pasta recipe.

This pasta dish is a midweek favourite in our household. It is one of those speedy pasta dishes where you can cook up the sauce in the time that it takes the pasta to cook. Quick, filling, sustaining, flavoursome and perfectly balanced with plenty of carbohydrate, heaps of vitamins and minerals from the greens, mushrooms and garlic and a little protein and fat from the eggs and bacon.

Nutrition per serving

Energy (kcal)	800	Protein (g)	34
Carbohydrate (g)	92	Fat (g)	36
Of which sugars (g)	8	Of which saturates (g)	16
Salt (g)	2.4	Fibre (g)	5

Serves 4
Prep time – 5 minutes/Cooking time – 10 minutes

450–500g spaghetti
400g spinach
8 rashers streaky bacon or a pack of lardons/pancetta cubes
250g mushrooms
1 small red chilli or a red pepper, deseeded and sliced finely
2 tbsp olive oil
300g low-fat crème fraîche
2 cloves of garlic, peeled and crushed
salt and pepper
¼ tsp grated nutmeg
50g grated parmesan, plus extra parmesan shavings to serve
4 eggs, lightly beaten

1. Cook the spaghetti according to instructions in plenty of salted water.
2. Meanwhile, gently fry the bacon, mushrooms and red chilli in olive oil for about 5 minutes. Add the crème fraîche and bring to a gentle simmer.

3. When the spaghetti is ready, drain it and then return it to the saucepan with a small ladleful of the cooking water.
4. Add the bacon, mushrooms and chilli and stir in the raw spinach and garlic.
5. On the lowest possible heat, add the parmesan, the seasoning and nutmeg and then, at the very last minute, turn off the heat and stir in the lightly beaten eggs.
6. Serve in big pasta bowls with extra shavings of parmesan and black pepper and a green salad with a lovely Dijon mustard dressing on the side.

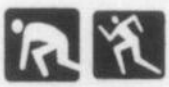

Tagliatelle with Walnuts

A nutritious and delicious pasta dish, good for the night before a big endurance session.

Walnuts are a great superfood. They are very high in omega-3 essential fatty acids and antioxidants. My parents have a walnut tree in their garden in France, so I am constantly trying to find uses for them. Unfortunately for me, that means I have to spend hours cracking them. However, it is much easier and just as healthy to buy them ready shelled. Try to use the fresh green spinach tagliatelle you can buy in most supermarkets.

Nutrition per serving

Energy (kcal)	591	Protein (g)	19
Carbohydrate (g)	78	Fat (g)	25
Of which sugars (g)	6	Of which saturates (g)	3.5
Salt (g)	0.4	Fibre (g)	5

Serves 4
Prep time – 2 minutes/Cooking time – 5–10 minutes

400g tagliatelle
1 tbsp olive oil
1 large shallot, chopped finely
1 clove of garlic, peeled and crushed
4 handfuls of walnuts, broken up but not chopped small
large bunch of flat-leaf parsley, chopped roughly
zest and juice of 1 lemon
2 tbsp extra virgin olive oil
salt and freshly ground black pepper
25g parmesan cheese, shaved

1. Preheat the oven to 160°C/gas mark 3.
2. Roast the walnuts in the oven for about 5 minutes. Be vigilant and watch that you don't burn them.
3. Cook the tagliatelle according to the pack instructions.

4. Meanwhile, gently fry the shallot in a large pan in a good tablespoon of olive oil. Add the garlic, walnuts, parsley and lemon zest.
5. When the pasta is cooked, drain, reserving a small ladleful of the cooking water, and transfer to the pan. Toss the pasta and the walnut mixture together. Add the cooking water and some tasty extra virgin olive oil to keep the mixture from becoming sticky.
6. Season with salt, black pepper, lemon juice and serve with a good helping of parmesan shavings.

Fazzoletti with Spring Vegetables and Fresh Herbs

Tasty vegetarian meal, rich in low-G.I. carbohydrate. Great for training and a nice alternative way of eating pasta.

'Fazzoletti', or 'handkerchiefs', are squares of lasagne pasta which are boiled and served with a sauce rather than baked in the oven. You simply layer the pasta and the sauce on the plate before serving. Yes, it is that easy! Cook the lasagne sheets, make the sauce and assemble on the plate. I like this recipe because it tastes super fresh and is very light. It is packed with vitamins yet it provides a good amount of carbohydrate and some protein from the sauce and the cheese. You can vary the vegetables you use, but it does look and taste best if you stick to green veg.

Nutrition per serving

Energy (kcal)	560	Protein (g)	20
Carbohydrate (g)	84	Fat (g)	18
Of which sugars (g)	9	Of which saturates (g)	7
Salt (g)	0.7	Fibre (g)	6.5

Serves 4
Prep time – 2 minutes/Cooking time – 10 minutes

12 fresh lasagne sheets
handful of peas
handful of broad beans, shelled
handful of French beans, trimmed
handful of asparagus (optional)
handful of fresh herbs (basil, parsley, chives or dill, or a mixture) chopped, plus extra to serve
25g unsalted butter
1 tbsp plain flour
300ml milk
splash of white wine
salt and pepper

pinch of grated nutmeg
pinch of paprika
tasty extra virgin olive oil or walnut oil
grated parmesan cheese to serve

1. Cook the lasagne sheets according to pack instructions. Warm a couple of plates.
2. Bring a pan of salted water to the boil and cook the vegetables for a minute or two – don't cook them for too long as they should have a slight crunch to them.
3. Drain the vegetables and put them aside. Make a béchamel sauce – gently melt the butter in a small pan, add the flour and stir vigorously to make a paste, cook on a low heat for a minute, add the milk gradually, stirring all the time, and cook until the sauce thickens a little (you don't want it too thick).
4. Add the white wine to the pan and boil gently for a couple of minutes. Season with some salt and pepper, a sprinkle of nutmeg and paprika, and then add the vegetables and the herbs. (If you prefer a sharper taste, use a small 300g pot of low-fat crème fraîche, a splash of wine and a knob of butter instead of the béchamel sauce.)
5. Pour a little of the olive or walnut oil onto each warmed plate and then, starting and ending with the lasagne, layer the lasagne and the sauce. Decorate with some herbs, parmesan and a drizzle of the olive or walnut oil.

Courgette Pasta Millefeuille with a Tomato Salad

A fresh-tasting, healthy, low-fat vegetarian meal. Light on the stomach, so a good meal to have before a training session.

Courgettes are delicious and easy to cook. They are low in calories with a good amount of vitamins A and C, plus folic acid and potassium. This is my healthy, endurance version of a millefeuille – a traditional cream cake made with layers of puff pastry and custard cream. I swap the layers of pastry with fresh lasagne sheets, and the custard cream with griddled courgettes, peppers, feta cheese and a basil dressing. Much easier to make, lower in fat and more sustaining. You can replace the courgettes with griddled aubergines if you like.

Nutrition per serving

Energy (kcal)	594	Protein (g)	20
Carbohydrate (g)	76	Fat (g)	25
Of which sugars (g)	18	Of which saturates (g)	8
Salt (g)	2	Fibre (g)	8

Serves 4
Prep time – 20 minutes (including cooking the vegetables)/ Cooking time – 5–10 mins

For the millefeuille

4 red peppers
5 or 6 medium-sized courgettes, sliced as thinly as possible lengthways using a sharp knife or a mandolin if you have one
2 tbsp olive oil
10 fresh lasagne sheets
bunch of fresh basil, chopped finely, plus some leaves for decoration.
3 tbsp good-quality, fruity olive oil
1 tbsp good-quality balsamic vinegar (white is preferable for this recipe)
squeeze of lemon juice
200g pack of feta cheese, sliced as thinly as possible
freshly ground black pepper

For the tomato salad

5–6 ripe vine tomatoes, sliced
1 mild onion, peeled and sliced as thinly as possible
about 8 black Kalamata olives, pitted if desired, and/or a tbsp of capers
good grind of black pepper and a sprinkling of sea salt
handful of basil leaves, torn up
squeeze of lemon juice
generous glug of good olive oil

1. Preheat the oven to 220°C/gas mark 7.
2. Mix all the tomato salad ingredients together, arrange on a plate and chill.
3. Put the red peppers into the hot oven for 15 minutes until blackened. Remove the peppers and leave to cool slightly (you can pop them into a plastic bag and leave them for 5 minutes if you like – the steam created makes the peel come off really easily), then peel, deseed and cut into quarters.
4. Heat a griddle or frying pan until really hot, brush the courgette strips with olive oil and cook in the rest of the oil for a couple of minutes on each side.
5. Meanwhile, bring a pan of salted water to the boil and cook the lasagne according to pack instructions, normally a couple of minutes. Cut the pasta sheets in half so that you have 20 sheets.
6. Chop the basil as small as possible and mix with the olive oil, lemon juice and vinegar.
7. Arrange layers of pasta, courgette and feta (the feta will crumble) and then peppers. Give each layer a drizzle of the basil dressing and a good grind of black pepper. Build up the layers so that each portion has about 5 sheets of pasta – 2 layers of courgette, 2 layers of peppers and one layer of pasta on the top.
8. Crumble some more feta and some basil leaves over the top and drizzle with the dressing.
9. Serve with the salad of fresh ripe tomatoes and eat with a sharp knife to cut cleanly through the lasagne sheets

Farfalle with Roasted Artichokes, Caramelised Leeks and Pine Nuts

Truly delicious low G.I. meal, good for endurance and pre-race carbo-loading.

These attractive bow-tie pasta shapes work extremely well with this combination of textures and flavours, and are perfect for a midweek carbohydrate-rich meal or for one of your meals in the days running up to a big race. You will find the marinated artichokes with the jars of antipasti in the supermarket.

Nutrition per serving

Energy (kcal)	499	Protein (g)	16
Carbohydrate (g)	78	Fat (g)	16
Of which sugars (g)	6	Of which saturates (g)	3
Salt (g)	0.1	Fibre (g)	5

Serves 4
Prep time – 5 minutes/Cooking time – 15 minutes

1 tbsp olive oil
knob of butter
1 large leek, sliced finely
400g farfalle
1 clove of garlic, peeled and finely sliced
1 dried chilli, crushed
zest of 1 lemon
200g marinated roasted artichokes, drained
handful of pine nuts
2 tbsp crème fraîche
freshly ground black pepper
1 tbsp chopped flat-leaved parsley (or 2 tsp pesto)
parmesan shavings to serve

1. Preheat the oven to 180°C/gas mark 4.
2. Heat the olive oil and butter in a non-stick frying pan. Add the

leeks and a sprinkling of brown sugar and fry gently for 10 minutes until they start to caramelise.

3. Bring a large saucepan of salted water to the boil and cook the farfalle according to pack instructions.
4. Add the garlic, chilli, lemon zest and artichokes to the leeks.
5. Meanwhile, roast the pine nuts in the oven for 5 minutes, until golden. Watch they don't burn!
6. Drain the pasta when it is cooked, carefully reserving a spoonful of the cooking liquid. Toss the pasta, cooking liquid and the leek and artichoke mixture together. Add the crème fraîche, pine nuts, plenty of black pepper and the parsley.
7. Serve on warmed pasta plates with plenty of parmesan shavings.

Farfalle with truffle oil and parmesan

Wonderful pre-exercise meal; light on the stomach, tasty, and high in slow-burning, low G.I. carbohydrate.

This really is the simplest pasta dish going, yet it is elegant and incredibly tasty. I was given a bottle of truffle oil as a gift recently and I have used it in this pasta, in a mushroom omelette and on a salad so far. The flavour is delicate and refined. Truffle oil is normally sold in delicatessens, although I have seen it on the shelf with the speciality oils in some supermarkets. An alternative would be a good quality walnut oil. Try it with any fresh pasta, such as fresh linguini, as well. It may sound odd, but a poached egg over the pasta is good if you fancy a bit of protein with your meal.

Nutrition per serving

Energy (kcal)	410	Protein (g)	15
Carbohydrate (g)	74	Fat (g)	8
Of which sugars (g)	3.5	Of which saturates (g)	2
Salt (g)	0.1	Fibre (g)	3.5

Serves 4
Prep time – a few minutes to heat up the pasta water/ Cooking time – 10 mins

400g farfalle
20ml truffle oil
20g fresh parmesan, shaved
freshly ground black pepper

1. Bring a large saucepan of salted water to the boil and cook the farfalle according to pack instructions.
2. When the pasta is al dente, drain it and pour it back into the saucepan. Pour in the truffle oil and mix it together.
3. Divide it between 4 warmed pasta bowls and sprinkle with parmesan shavings and black pepper.
4. Delicious served with a salad of green beans.

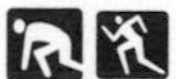

Lemon Basil Spaghetti

Very good pre-exercise lunch – light on the stomach but sustaining and full of goodness.

This is simple, tasty, healthy fast food. Packed with good, slow-burning carbohydrate, vitamin C from the lemon, basil and garlic and a little protein and calcium from the cheese, this dish is fantastic as a starter or as a light, summery lunch. Basil also contains high levels of calcium and vitamin K, both important bone-building nutrients. This spaghetti is also delicious with fresh tarragon instead of basil.

Nutrition per serving

Energy (kcal)	352	Protein (g)	12
Carbohydrate (g)	56	Fat (g)	9
Of which sugars (g)	3	Of which saturates (g)	2
Salt (g)	0.2	Fibre (g)	2.5

Makes 4 medium portions
Prep time – 2–3 minutes/Cooking time – 10 minutes

300g spaghetti (wholemeal or white)
2 tbsp lemon juice
zest of 1 unwaxed lemon
2 tbsp extra virgin olive oil
4 tbsp white wine
1 clove of garlic, peeled and crushed
plenty of freshly ground black pepper
large handful of fresh basil leaves, torn, plus a few for decoration.
25g freshly grated parmesan

1. Cook the spaghetti in plenty of salted boiling water according to pack instructions.
2. While the spaghetti is cooking, combine all the ingredients except the parmesan and gently warm in a saucepan.
3. When the spaghetti is cooked, drain it reserving a spoonful of the cooking liquid and combine with the lemon basil sauce.
4. Serve with extra fresh basil leaves, black pepper and parmesan.

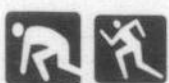

Linguini with Cavolo Nero and Lardons

This is a tasty and easy weekday pasta dish to include in your training programme.

Cavolo nero is an Italian cabbage, fairly widely available in the UK now. It is a beautiful plant and personally I think that it looks good enough to give as a bunch of flowers. It has lustrous dark green leaves and a strong, buttery flavour and it is *really* healthy, containing vitamins K, A and C, B vitamins and fibre as well as minerals such as manganese, iron, calcium and copper. I love it.

Nutrition per serving

Energy (kcal)	690	Protein (g)	24
Carbohydrate (g)	80	Fat (g)	33
Of which sugars (g)	9	Of which saturates (g)	12
Salt (g)	3	Fibre (g)	5

Serves 4
Prep time – 5 minutes/Cooking time – 15 minutes

400g linguini, wholewheat or standard
250g bunch of cavolo nero, chopped roughly
250g lardons or cubed pancetta or bacon
1 red pepper, deseeded and sliced
½ tbsp oil to sauté
1 clove of garlic, peeled and crushed
1 anchovy fillet, chopped
2 tbsp crème fraîche
a splash of milk
salt and plenty of black pepper
glug of extra virgin olive oil
parmesan shavings to serve

1. Cook the cavolo nero gently in a large pan, covered, in about 1cm of water or steam in a steamer. It should be wilted and tender – this will take about 5 minutes.

2. In a large non-stick frying pan, sauté the lardons and red pepper in the oil until the bacon is cooked and the pepper is soft.
3. Cook the linguini in plenty of salted boiling water according to the instructions on the pack.
4. When the cavolo nero is tender, remove it from the pan with a slotted spoon and add it to the pan with the lardons. Add the garlic, anchovy, crème fraîche and a splash of milk and simmer gently for a couple of minutes.
5. Drain the pasta, reserving a little of the cooking liquid, and add the pasta to the pan with the lardons mixture. Add plenty of salt and freshly ground black pepper and combine everything together with a little of the cooking liquid from the pasta.
6. Finally pour over a glug of olive oil – it will go deliciously glossy – finish with a shaving of parmesan and serve.

Linguini with Mussels, Chilli, White Wine and Crème Fraîche

Excellent source of iron and good for endurance training.

This dish is equally good with fresh clams, which, along with mussels, are high in iron. Iron levels get depleted during hard exercise so it is really important to keep them topped up, especially if you are a woman. Preparing the mussels may seem a bit of a chore, but it only takes 10 minutes and can be quite therapeutic.

Nutrition per serving

Energy (kcal)	700	Protein (g)	35
Carbohydrate (g)	95	Fat (g)	28
Of which sugars (g)	7	Of which saturates (g)	12
Salt (g)	0.9	Fibre (g)	4

Serves 4
Prep time – 10–15 minutes/Cooking time – 15 minutes

500g linguini
1½kg mussels
225ml white wine
bunch of fresh flat-leaved parsley, roughly chopped
2 large cloves of garlic, peeled and crushed
2 dried chillies, chopped small
lots of freshly ground black pepper
300ml crème fraîche
extra virgin olive oil
salt to taste

1. Prepare the mussels – under running water, scrub them and pull off any stringy beards sticking out from them. Discard any mussels that do not close up when you clean them.
2. Bring a large pan of water to the boil for the linguine.
3. Place the mussels in a large pan with a tight-fitting lid, with the wine, half the parsley, the garlic, chilli and pepper and cook on a

high heat for about five minutes, with the lid tightly on. Shake them or stir them during that time so that the mussels at the top get the chance to cook in the juice at the bottom.

4. After about 5 minutes, when the mussels are cooked (they will have opened and will start to look plump), turn off the heat. If you can be bothered, take about half of them out of their shells. Discard any that haven't opened.
5. Cook the linguini according to the instructions on the pack. Drain and then pop back into the pan, with a small ladle of the cooking liquid. Keep on a very low heat, add the crème fraîche, the mussels and all their juice (check that there is no grit in the mussel juice – if there is you'll need to strain it). Taste and season.
6. Throw in the rest of the parsley and then a really decent glug of fruity extra virgin olive oil.
7. This linguini looks fantastic presented at the table in one large serving dish. You could put some extra chilli in a small bowl for people to sprinkle on top, if you like.

Pappardelle with Scallops, Broad Beans, Bacon and Mint

Low-G.I. dish with a high percentage of carbohydrate – quick to make and perfect for training.

This is one of my store cupboard recipes, hence the use of frozen scallops and broad beans, which I tend to keep in the freezer just in case. I love being able to knock up a delicious and healthy dish without having to shop specially, but by all means use fresh produce if you like. Pappardelle are wide, flat ribbons of pasta, which are fantastic if you can get them fresh. Otherwise use the dried version, or any other robust pasta, like tagliatelle or torn up lasagne sheets. The flavours in this pasta just seem to complement each other perfectly. Scallops are really good for you, containing vitamin B12, omega-3 fatty acids, magnesium and potassium, nutrients which are excellent for cardiovascular health.

Nutrition per serving

Energy (kcal)	597	Protein (g)	29
Carbohydrate (g)	71	Fat (g)	24
Of which sugars (g)	3	Of which saturates (g)	9
Salt (g)	2.2	Fibre (g)	6

Serves 4
Prep time – 5 minutes/Cooking time – 10 minutes

360g pappardelle, fresh if you can
200g fresh or frozen broad beans
100g lardons or bacon pieces
½ tsp oil for frying
200g pack of frozen scallops, or 12–16 fresh, cleaned and patted dry with a cloth
large handful of fresh mint leaves, chopped
salt and plenty of black pepper
2 tbsp crème fraîche
100g feta cheese, very thinly cut into slivers

1. Cook the pappardelle according to the pack instructions in a large saucepan with plenty of salted water.
2. Cook the broad beans for a couple of minutes in boiling salted water. Drain them and peel off the outer skins.
3. Heat a large frying pan and fry the bacon pieces in ½ tsp of oil. Keep the heat up high and add the frozen scallops. Fry them for about 3 minutes on each side. By this time, the scallops will be just cooked through and caramelised on the outside and the bacon will be nice and crispy. If you use fresh scallops, you will only need to cook them for a minute or so each side.
4. Add the broad beans, the chopped mint, reserving some to sprinkle on top later, and plenty of black pepper.
5. When the pappardelle is ready, drain and combine with the broad bean mixture. Add the crème fraîche and serve on warmed pasta in bowls with the slivers of feta cheese and more fresh mint sprinkled on top.

Scallop and Chorizo Trofie

Surprise your non-sporty friends with this absolutely delicious dish which is actually perfectly nutritionally balanced for training or for a pre-race meal.

Pasta day in, day out, can become really quite monotonous. However, it is still one of the best ways to get good carbohydrate into our bodies, so take the opportunity to be a bit adventurous. Trofie can be bought in the speciality pasta section of the supermarket. They are quite delicious tossed with this mixture of sweet, succulent scallops and spicy chorizo. If you can afford them, use good-quality ingredients – fresh diver-caught scallops, good olive oil and balsamic vinegar and a glass of Sauvignon Blanc.

Nutrition per serving

Energy (kcal)	574	Protein (g)	25
Carbohydrate (g)	72	Fat (g)	20
Of which sugars (g)	4.5	Of which saturates (g)	1
Salt (g)	1.9	Fibre (g)	4

Serves 4
Prep time – 10 minutes/Cooking time – 15 minutes

350–400g trofie pasta
salt and freshly ground black pepper
100g spicy chorizo sausage, sliced into ½cm coins
1 large green pepper, deseeded and cut into slices
1 small clove of garlic, peeled and crushed
large handful of fresh flat-leaf parsley, chopped, plus some extra leaves to serve
2 tbsp extra virgin olive oil
12 scallops (fresh if possible)
225ml fruity white wine
1 tbsp good-quality balsamic vinegar
pinch of Spanish smoked paprika

1. Bring a large saucepan of salted water to boil and cook the trofie according to the instructions on the pack – usually about 12 minutes. Put four plates or pasta bowls in the oven to warm.
2. Prepare the scallops – trim them and slice each in half horizontally so that you get two circles. Dry them with some kitchen towel and sprinkle them with a little salt and pepper.
3. Heat a non-stick frying pan and, when it is hot, dry fry the chorizo until the fat starts to run out. Turn over the chorizo slices so that they crisp up on both sides, then add the green peppers and sauté these for a couple of minutes – not too much as you want them to be quite crunchy. Turn the heat down and then add the garlic and sauté for 30 seconds or so (don't let the garlic burn).
4. When the trofie is cooked, drain it, pop it back in the saucepan and add the chorizo/pepper mix (leaving a little of the oil from the chorizo in the frying pan) and the parsley and mix together with the extra virgin olive oil. Turn this mixture out onto the warmed plates.
5. Heat the frying pan again and when it is really hot add the scallops and fry them on a high heat for about 30 seconds each side.
6. Divide the scallops between the 4 plates.
7. Pour a small glass of wine and a scant tbsp of balsamic vinegar into the frying pan and let it bubble away, scraping any caramelised bits from the bottom of the frying pan. Pour a little over each portion.
8. Scatter with some parsley leaves and a sprinkling of smoked paprika (use normal paprika if you don't have any) and a little black pepper. Eat immediately.

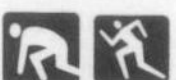

Spaghetti with Fresh Herbs

Ideal for endurance: a good source of low-G.I. carbohydrate, light on the stomach with plenty of vitamins from the herbs and garlic, plus a little protein from the cheese. Anchovies are high in sodium, so adding these is a really good way of naturally increasing salt intake if you lose a lot through sweat.

Sometimes the simplest things are the best. In Italy, pasta with fresh herbs is cooked as a staple dish, rather like beans on toast in Britain! Good herbs to use are flat-leaf parsley, basil, chives, mint, marjoram, oregano ... whatever you can lay your hands on.

Nutrition per serving

Energy (kcal)	506	Protein (g)	18
Carbohydrate (g)	75	Fat (g)	17
Of which sugars (g)	4	Of which saturates (g)	3
Salt (g)	1.1	Fibre (g)	5

Serves 4
Prep time – 5 minutes/Cooking time – 10 minutes

400g spaghetti (fresh, dried, standard or wholewheat)
4 tbsp extra virgin olive oil
2 cloves of garlic, peeled and crushed
1 dried chilli, crushed or a small fresh red chilli, deseeded and finely chopped
4 canned anchovy fillets, chopped small (optional)
grated zest of 1 lemon
100–150g fresh herbs (see above), chopped
freshly ground black pepper
grated parmesan cheese to serve

1. Bring a large pan of salted water to the boil and cook the spaghetti according to pack instructions.
2. In a large non-stick frying pan, sweat the garlic in the olive oil over a low heat for a minute and then add the chilli, lemon zest, anchovies and herbs and soften slightly.

3. Drain the spaghetti when it is cooked, reserving some of the cooking liquid to prevent the pasta from sticking together. Add the spaghetti to the herby sauce and toss well to combine. If you are not using anchovies, you may need to add some salt at this stage.
4. Serve with some parmesan cheese and freshly ground black pepper. A fresh tomato and basil salad goes really well with this dish as an accompaniment.

rice

'I found your information regarding G.I. levels very interesting and athletes will take note of this in their preparation. My favourite? Thai green fish curry [with rice noodles]!' Nick Rose, two-time Olympian and holder of the British record for the Half Marathon – 1:01:03.

'I never realised that rice was good for carbo-loading. After relying on the traditional, and deeply uninspiring, Spaghetti Bolognese for several years I think it's time for a change.' Andrew Shelling, solicitor, marathon and ultra marathon runner. Personal goal – to run the five world major marathons and complete the Biel 100km five times.

'Stuck for supper ideas again, I tried the saffron rice. Everyone agreed it was delicious; lovely subtle flavours and it seemed to serve hubby well on his 15 miler the next morning!' Julie McCarthy, patient and supportive marathon wife.

Creamy Risotto of Broad Beans, Mint and Pancetta

Relatively high-G.I., low-fat meal – good for recovery after a big workout.

This is one of my favourite risottos and is a great meal to eat straight after a marathon or a big endurance run, partly because it is easy and relaxing to make, partly because it has a relatively high G.I. factor: risotto rice has a G.I. of 69, the broad beans have a G.I. of 79. I ate this risotto in an Italian restaurant in Amsterdam after the Amsterdam Marathon and I am sure the carbohydrate shot straight to my tired muscles. If I am having a vegetarian moment, I make it without the pancetta. It is also delicious if you add 50g frozen or fresh peas.

Nutrition per serving

Energy (kcal)	730	Protein (g)	27
Carbohydrate (g)	88	Fat (g)	28
Of which sugars (g)	3.5	Of which saturates (g)	10
Salt (g)	2.4	Fibre (g)	6

Serves 4
Prep time – 10 minutes/Cooking time – 20–25 minutes

3 tbsp olive oil or 50g unsalted butter, plus a knob of butter for the end
1 onion, peeled and finely sliced
1 stick of celery, finely chopped
1 clove of garlic, peeled and crushed
80g pancetta cubes, or bacon, cubed
350g Arborio risotto rice
1¼–1½ litres vegetable bouillon or chicken stock
250ml white wine
300g broad beans, shelled (remove outer layer of beans if they are tough), or a pack of frozen broad beans
large bunch of fresh mint, chopped
100g freshly grated parmesan
salt and freshly ground black pepper

1. Heat up the stock in a saucepan so that it is ready to ladle onto the rice.
2. In a large heavy-bottomed pan, gently sauté the onion and celery in the butter/oil over a low heat until translucent. Add the garlic and the pancetta and sauté for another couple of minutes, without allowing it to brown.
3. Add the rice and stir until the grains become translucent and glossy.
4. Add the wine and stir until it has been absorbed.
5. Add a ladle of hot stock and stir constantly until it is almost absorbed. Add the rest of the hot stock, a ladle at a time, stirring constantly. You need to make sure that each ladleful is absorbed by the rice before you add the next one. This should take about 18–20 minutes. You may need more or less stock according to the type of rice and the rate of absorption.
6. When the rice is almost cooked, add the broad beans and the mint (save a little to sprinkle over the top). The texture should be nice and creamy. You may need to add some salt at this point, it depends how salty your stock is.
7. When the rice is cooked, turn off the heat, stir in the parmesan and a knob of butter. Let the mixture stand for a couple of minutes. Sprinkle with the remaining mint and a few grinds of black pepper.
8. Serve with a rocket salad and some fresh parmesan shavings.

Duck, Orange and Cardamom Pilaf

Low G.I., great for endurance, tastes exotic but is dead easy to make.

When you finally lift the lid off this pilaf, the beautiful aroma just blows you away. Perfect for endurance, this pilaf is light and fluffy and feels like quite a treat. The fact is it only takes about 30 minutes to make and you can buy packets of Gressingham duck legs in the supermarkets at a very reasonable price nowadays. My French friends insist that duck is good for you. It is high in protein and an important source of iron, and the fat is lower in saturated fat and cholesterol than butter. The whole family loves this dish, but I particularly like to cook it to keep up my and my daughter's iron levels.

Nutrition per serving

Energy (kcal)	760	Protein (g)	50
Carbohydrate (g)	106	Fat (g)	18
Of which sugars (g)	18	Of which saturates (g)	4
Salt (g)	1.3	Fibre (g)	2

Serves 4
Prep time – 5 minutes/Cooking time – 35 minutes

4 duck legs (ideally Gressingham)
1½ tsp allspice
½ tsp cardamom powder
½ tsp salt
1 tsp oil for frying
1 onion, peeled and sliced finely
1 bay leaf
12 cardamom pods, crushed lightly with a pestle and mortar
freshly ground black pepper
1 cinnamon stick
400g basmati rice, rinsed a couple of times and then drained
3–4 tbsp currants
juice and zest of 1 orange

600ml chicken stock
salt
handful of flaked almonds, toasted
handful of finely chopped fresh mint or coriander

1. Trim off any excess skin and fat from the duck legs with some scissors, pat them dry and then sprinkle them with ½ tsp of the allspice, and the cardamom powder and salt.
2. Heat the oil in a non-stick frying pan and gently fry the duck legs, skin side down, for about 10 minutes, until the skin is good and crisp. Turn them over and continue to cook gently for another 10 minutes or so until cooked through. Spoon off the fat every now and then and reserve (kept in the fridge, it is perfect for roast potatoes).
3. Meanwhile, heat a couple of tablespoons of the fat in a saucepan (make sure you use one with a tight-fitting lid) and gently sauté the onion until it is translucent. Add the remaining allspice, cardamom pods, black pepper, bay leaf and cinnamon stick and stir for a minute or two to release the aromas.
4. Add the rice and stir it around so that it becomes glossy. Stir in the currants and orange zest and then add the stock, the orange juice and some salt (the amount will depend how salty your stock is).
5. Quickly bring the stock to the boil, turn down to a very low heat, place a circle of greaseproof paper over the liquid and cover with the tight-fitting lid.
6. Cook on the lowest heat for 7 minutes and then turn off the heat and leave, still covered, for a further 7 minutes. Remove the lid, enjoy the aroma and test for seasoning.
7. By this time the duck should be cooked. Spoon off the fat and scrape any juices from the duck pan to drizzle over the rice. Arrange the pilaf with the crispy duck onto a large hot serving dish or four individual plates. Scatter over the almonds and the coriander or mint.

Green Chicken Curry

diet – low in fat, low G.I., packed with

...of a very quick and easy Indian chicken curry. ...most creamy Indian curries, this one is pretty low fat, made with low-fat yoghurt and skinless chicken thighs. You just whiz up the sauce in a blender and cook it with the chicken. Because of the large amount of fresh coriander and mint, the sauce is a vibrant green and is packed with vitamin C and antioxidants. The ginger, a great source of minerals such as potassium, copper, manganese and vitamin B6, is said to be an anti-inflammatory and can help towards muscle repair. My children love this so my version is relatively mild – by all means add some more green chilli if you would like a bit more heat. If you eat this with a good portion of basmati rice (brown or white) it should provide you with a really healthy meal which will help towards endurance. We love this with naan bread too.

Nutrition per serving

Energy (kcal)	614	Protein (g)	31
Carbohydrate (g)	98	Fat (g)	13
Of which sugars (g)	9	Of which saturates (g)	3
Salt (g)	1.4	Fibre (g)	2.5

Serves 4
Prep time – 5 minutes/Cooking time – 25 minutes

350g low-fat natural yoghurt
90g (large bunch) fresh coriander – leaves and stalks
25g fresh mint leaves
20g (or 3cm lump) fresh ginger, peeled and chopped roughly
3–4 cloves of garlic, peeled and roughly chopped
2 green chillies, chopped, with seeds remaining
1 onion, peeled and chopped
1 tbsp sunflower oil

8 skinless, boneless chicken thighs, fat trimmed off
2 heaped tsp ground coriander
6 cardamom pods, bruised in a pestle and mortar
1 tsp ground cumin
½–1 tsp salt
400g basmati rice
toasted flaked almonds and chopped mint leaves to serve

1. Start by putting the yoghurt, the fresh herbs, the ginger, garlic, chilli and onion into a blender and puree until you get a smooth, bright green sauce.
2. Heat a large non-stick pan (with a lid). When it is hot, add the oil and brown the chicken over a high heat for a few minutes.
3. Pour in the sauce and turn the chicken so that it is coated with the sauce. Add the ground coriander, cardamom and cumin and cook on a high heat for 2 minutes.
4. Cover and simmer for about 20 minutes (you might need 5 minutes longer if the chicken is on the bone).
5. Meanwhile cook the rice according to pack instructions.
6. Remove the lid, add salt to taste. Test the chicken is cooked through by cutting into a piece with a sharp knife to ensure that the meat is no longer pink.
7. Serve immediately. Sprinkle some almonds and mint leaves on top for decoration. I also put a bowl of freshly chopped green chilli on the table to sprinkle over.

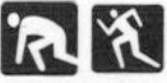

Moorish Lamb Kebabs on a Bed of Saffron Rice with Dried Cranberries, Cardamom and Pistachios

Excellent balanced, healthy low-fat meal, good for training but equally good enough for a late summer supper party.

This dish always reminds me of summer evenings in the garden. Our great British weather can sometimes dictate otherwise and these evenings can be few and far between, so luckily these kebabs are just as good cooked on a griddle or under the grill inside. They are delicious served with a quickly made yoghurt sauce, some chilli sauce or harissa. The basmati rice is a good low-G.I. option for your training and the dried fruit, nuts and spices not only add vital nutrients, but also a taste of the sun. You can use brown or white basmati rice for this dish and if you do not have time to soak the rice, make sure you rinse it well until the water is clear and cook it for a little longer. If you want to reduce the fat content of this recipe, just use less butter in the rice.

Nutrition per serving

Energy (kcal)	880	Protein (g)	44
Carbohydrate (g)	64	Fat (g)	52
Of which sugars (g)	10	Of which saturates (g)	23
Salt (g)	1.7	Fibre (g)	1

Serves 4 (8 kebabs)
Prep time – 10 minutes + marinating/
Cooking time – 15 minutes (cook kebabs and rice at same time)
You will need 8 skewers (if these are bamboo, see step 2)

For the rice
100g unsalted butter
1 x 5cm cinnamon stick
6 cardamom pods, crushed
2 bay leaves

4 black peppercorns, crushed
250g basmati rice – soaked for 2–3 hours, then rinsed and drained
50g pistachio nuts
handful of dried cranberries (use raisins or chopped apricots as an alternative)
pinch of dried saffron, soaked in a few tbsp of boiling water and left for 10 minutes to infuse (if you have no saffron, use a pinch of turmeric instead – you don't need to soak this)
salt
freshly chopped coriander and mint to sprinkle on top

For the kebabs
3 tbsp olive oil
juice and zest of 1 lemon
2 cloves of garlic, roughly crushed
2 tsp cumin seeds, roughly ground
2 tsp coriander seeds, roughly ground
1 tsp sweet smoked paprika
salt and freshly ground pepper
700g lamb fillet or boneless lamb leg, cubed

For the yoghurt sauce
200g low-fat natural yoghurt
1 clove of garlic, peeled and crushed
pinch of salt and freshly ground back pepper
25g bunch fresh mint leaves, finely chopped

1. To make the kebabs, place the cubes of lamb into a mixing bowl and add the marinade ingredients. Leave overnight or as long as you can for the flavours to infuse.
2. If you are using bamboo skewers, soak them into a bowl of water for ½ hour or so before using – otherwise they will burn.
3. Thread the meat onto your kebab sticks. Keep the marinade for basting.
4. Heat the griddle or grill so that it is really hot and cook the kebabs for about 10–15 minutes, turning and basting with the marinade

every few minutes, until crisp and brown on the outside and slightly pink on the inside.

5. To make the rice, melt the butter in a large saucepan and add the cinnamon stick, cardamom pods, bay leaves and crushed black peppercorns. Gently sauté over a low heat for a few minutes until the spice aromas start to be released.
6. Add the rice and stir gently to coat it in the butter.
7. Add the pistachios, cranberries and saffron water then pour enough water to cover the rice by about 1cm. Add some salt at this stage. Bring to the boil, cover tightly and simmer very gently for 10 minutes, or until the rice is cooked. If you use brown basmati rice, you will need a longer cooking time.
8. To make the yoghurt sauce, mix together the yoghurt and garlic with a pinch of salt, some freshly ground black pepper and the mint.
9. Serve the rice on a large platter with the kebabs piled on top and sprinkle generously with the chopped coriander and mint. Serve the yoghurt sauce separately in a bowl as an accompaniment.

Pink Peppercorn Risotto with Pork and Peanuts

Great to eat after a heavy exercise session; warming and nutritious and a perfect opportunity to do your stretches while you are stirring the risotto.

Pink peppercorns seem to go really well with pork and they give this risotto a truly exceptional flavour. You can buy them in supermarkets or delicatessens either dried or, better still, in little jars of brine. They give this risotto a deliciously aromatic flavour. You can use the same method with basmati rice rather than risotto rice if you fancy a pilau rather than a risotto.

Nutrition per serving

Energy (kcal)	657	Protein (g)	42
Carbohydrate (g)	82	Fat (g)	18
Of which sugars (g)	4	Of which saturates (g)	5
Salt (g)	0.8	Fibre (g)	2.5

Serves 4
Prep time – 5 minutes/Cooking time – 20–25 minutes

15g unsalted butter plus a tbsp oil
1 onion, peeled and sliced finely
1 leek, sliced finely
1 stick celery, chopped finely
2 medium pork tenderloins (about 700g), trimmed of any fat and cut into ½cm rounds
350g risotto rice such as arborio or vialone nano
225ml glass of white wine or sherry
1¼–1½ litres hot chicken stock
1 tbsp pink peppercorns, crushed a little with a pestle and mortar
1 clove of garlic, peeled and crushed
1 tsp ground ginger
handful of salted peanuts
handful of fresh coriander

1. Heat up the stock in a saucepan so that it is ready to ladle onto the rice.
2. In a large heavy-bottomed pan, gently sauté the onion, leek and celery in the butter/oil over a low heat until translucent. Add the pork and cook for a couple of minutes to seal it.
3. Add the rice and stir until the grains become translucent and glossy.
4. Add the glass of wine and stir constantly until it is absorbed. Add a ladle of hot stock and again stir until it is completely absorbed. Continue to add the hot stock, a ladle at a time. You need to make sure that each ladleful is absorbed by the rice before you add the next one. This should take about 18–20 minutes. You may need more or less stock according to the type of rice and the rate of absorption.
5. When the rice is almost cooked, add the pink peppercorns, the garlic, the ginger, half the peanuts and the coriander (save a little to sprinkle over the top).You may need to add some salt at this point, it depends how salty your stock is. Stir it all round and then leave it to rest for a couple of minutes.
6. Sprinkle with the remaining coriander and the rest of the peanuts.

Quick Seafood Paella

Good for recovery – a great balance of carbohydrate, protein, vitamins, iron and other minerals.

This delicious Spanish paella is very easy to make, excellent for training and is a complete balanced meal in one dish. If you can't get to the fishmonger you can use frozen seafood quite successfully, just use what is available. Spanish paella rice is a short-grain rice, which is a relatively high-G.I. carbohydrate. This means that it is digested quickly into your system and therefore very good to eat if you have just had an intensive workout as it will help your muscles recover as quickly as possible. To make this dish more suitable for endurance, just use a low-G.I. basmati rice instead and add a can of chickpeas or butter beans at stage 4 of the cooking. Try to buy a spicy chorizo in its whole 'sausage' form rather than sliced – it is usually in a pack on the shelf with other prepacked whole salamis in the supermarket.

Nutrition per serving

Energy (kcal)	783	Protein (g)	47
Carbohydrate (g)	96	Fat (g)	26
Of which sugars (g)	5	Of which saturates (g)	2
Salt (g)	3.7	Fibre (g)	3

Serves 4

Prep time – 10 minutes if using fresh seafood, less if frozen/ Cooking time – 25 minutes

4 chicken thighs, bone in (free-range is best if you can afford them)
2 tbsp olive oil
1 large onion, peeled and sliced
1 red pepper, deseeded and sliced
2 bay leaves
4 cloves of garlic, peeled and crushed
2 tsp paprika (preferably smoked Spanish paprika)
½ tsp cayenne pepper

½ jar sugocasa (use 400g tin of chopped tomatoes as an alternative)
400g Spanish paella rice
1 litre hot chicken stock with a pinch of saffron (include a glass of dry white wine in this amount if you like)
150g chorizo (spicy if possible, cut into large chunks)
large handful of frozen petit pois or peas
12 mussels, cleaned (wash under cold water, pull out the beard and discard any that do not close when you handle them)
12 large prawns in their shells
300g squid, cleaned and sliced
bunch of flat-leaf parsley, roughly chopped
lemon wedges to serve

1. Season the chicken and then brown it in a tbsp of oil in a really large frying pan or paella dish.
2. Remove the chicken pieces and then add the onion, bay leaf and red pepper. Sauté gently until the onion is golden.
3. Add the garlic, paprika, cayenne pepper and sugocasa and cook for a couple of minutes to release the aromas.
4. Add the rice and stir around so that the rice is nice and glossy.
5. Add the hot stock, the chicken and the chorizo, stir and cook gently, uncovered, without stirring, for 10 minutes. Shake the pan every now and then to stop the rice sticking.
6. Taste for seasoning – depending on the saltiness of your stock, you may need to add some salt. Stir in the peas and the mussels and cook for about another 10 minutes, without stirring, until the rice is cooked and the mussels have opened. You may need to add a little extra stock.
7. Heat the rest of the oil in a separate pan and quickly fry the prawns at a high heat until they turn pink, then add the squid and continue frying for a minute or two until the squid turns translucent. Add this to the paella, scraping out any juices.
8. Stir in the parsley, leave the paella to rest for a couple of minutes, place the pan on the table and serve with some lemon wedges to squeeze over. This tastes good with a green salad.

Three Grain Rice Risotto with Mushrooms

Good for carbo-loading the night before a race – easy to digest and sustaining.

The nutty flavour of this three grain rice is absolutely delicious. It is available in most supermarkets and is a mixture of risotto rice, spelt and barley. I buy Riso Gallo 3 Grains, but there are other brands around. Spelt is an ancient variety of wheat which is rich in protein and fibre. Along with the barley, it has a really low G.I., is easy to digest and has a lovely chewy, nutty texture. This risotto is a nice alternative if you are starting to tire of the standard carbohydrate fare towards the end of your training schedule. It is a really good meal to eat the night before a long training session. If I feel I need to up my protein and iron intake, I might serve this up alongside some delicious organic sausages, a rare, juicy piece of griddled steak or a roast chicken and a green salad.

Nutrition per serving

Energy (kcal)	570	Protein (g)	17
Carbohydrate (g)	81	Fat (g)	19
Of which sugars (g)	4	Of which saturates (g)	9
Salt (g)	1.6	Fibre (g)	3

Serves 4
Prep time – 5 minutes/Cooking time – 20 minutes

2 knobs of butter
1 tbsp olive oil
1 onion, peeled and finely sliced
1 leek, finely sliced
1 stick celery, finely chopped
2 cloves garlic, peeled and crushed
350g 3 grain rice
225ml white wine
1¼–1½ litres hot vegetable or chicken stock (include the mushroom soaking water, if using dried mushrooms)

250g mixed mushrooms – include chestnut mushrooms and field mushrooms, sliced, and porcini (use a pack of dried porcini and reconstitute in warm water)
1 tsp ground cumin
salt and plenty of freshly ground black pepper
large handful of fresh parsley or coriander, chopped
75g freshly grated parmesan, plus some extra for adding at the table

1. Heat up the stock in a saucepan so that it is ready to ladle onto the rice.
2. In a large heavy-bottomed pan, over a low heat, gently sauté the onion, leek and celery in the butter and oil until translucent. Add the garlic and gently sauté for a couple of minutes, without allowing it to brown.
3. Add the rice and stir until the grains become translucent and glossy. Add the glass of wine and stir constantly until it is absorbed. Add the hot stock, a ladle at a time. You need to make sure that each ladleful is absorbed by the rice before you add the next one. This should take about 18–20 minutes. You may need more or less stock according to the rate of absorption of the rice. After about 10 minutes, add the mushrooms and combine well with the rice.
4. When the rice is almost cooked, add the cumin, black pepper and the fresh herbs (save some to sprinkle over the top). The texture should be nice and creamy. You may need to add some salt at this point, it depends how salty your stock is.
5. When the rice is cooked, turn off the heat, stir in the parmesan and a knob of butter. Let the mixture stand for a couple of minutes. Sprinkle with the remaining herbs and a few grinds of black pepper.
6. Serve with extra grated parmesan to sprinkle over the top.

Roasted Butternut Squash Risotto with Maple Syrup Almonds

This is a wonderful midweek training dish for the autumn.

Butternut squash is one of those vegetables that has an amazing array of nutrients – it is an excellent source of the antioxidant and anti-inflammatory beta-carotene (vitamin A), it contains good amounts of vitamin C, potassium and fibre, plus folic acid, omega-3 fatty acids, vitamin B1, copper, niacin ... the list is endless. Add the almonds, parmesan and the risotto rice to this and you have a very tasty and nutritious low-G.I. meal. You can develop this meal into a higher G.I. recovery meal by replacing the butternut squash with pumpkin.

Nutrition per serving

Energy (kcal)	689	Protein (g)	18
Carbohydrate (g)	104	Fat (g)	22
Of which sugars (g)	12	Of which saturates (g)	8
Salt (g)	1.7	Fibre (g)	4

Serves 4

Prep time – 2 minutes/Cooking time – 25 minutes

1 butternut squash, peeled, seeds removed and cut into 2cm cubes
2 tbsp olive oil
1 tsp salt
freshly ground black pepper
2 knobs of butter
1 onion, peeled and finely sliced
1 clove of garlic, peeled and crushed
350g risotto rice – vialone nano or arborio
225ml dry white wine
1¼–1½ litres hot vegetable or chicken stock
small handful of flaked almonds
1 tbsp maple syrup, diluted with a few drops of water
1 tsp saffron strands (optional)
75g freshly grated parmesan

1. Preheat the oven to 200°C/gas mark 6.
2. Put the squash on a baking sheet and toss it with 1 tbsp olive oil, then sprinkle a tsp of salt and some freshly ground pepper over the top. Roast in the oven for about 25 minutes until the squash is tender and golden. Stir it once or twice while it is roasting.
3. Heat up the stock in a saucepan so that it is ready to ladle onto the rice.
4. Melt the butter and remaining olive oil in a large heavy-bottomed pan and gently sauté the onion until it becomes translucent. Add the garlic and gently sauté for a couple of minutes, without allowing it to brown.
5. Add the rice and stir until the grains become translucent and glossy.
6. Add the wine and cook for a couple of minutes until completely absorbed. If you are using saffron, stir it in now and then add the hot stock, a ladle at a time, otherwise just start with the stock. You need to make sure that each ladleful of stock is absorbed by the rice before you add the next one. This should take about 18–20 minutes. You may need more or less stock according to the type of rice and the rate of absorption.
7. Meanwhile mix the almonds with the maple syrup and water and pop them in the oven for about 5 minutes until golden.
8. The rice is cooked when it is slightly al dente and looks nice and creamy. Taste it to see if you need more salt (it depends how salty your stock is as to how much you need), turn off the heat, stir in the parmesan and the butternut squash and a generous knob of butter. Let the mixture stand for a couple of minutes.
9. Serve with the almonds and some fresh parmesan shavings.
10. This goes really well with a crisp salad (frisée or gem) with crispy bacon/pancetta pieces, tossed in a light balsamic dressing.

Roasted Salmon with Saffron Risotto

Perfect as a healthy midweek dish to brighten up your training diet.

Saffron risotto can be rustled up in a flash and yet it tastes very sophisticated. As an accompaniment to a piece of roasted salmon and some green beans, it can turn a simple meal into a very healthy, balanced, sustaining and delicious feast.

Nutrition per serving

Energy (kcal)	600	Protein (g)	27
Carbohydrate (g)	69	Fat (g)	23
Of which sugars (g)	4.5	Of which saturates (g)	8.5
Salt (g)	1	Fibre (g)	1

Serves 4
Prep time – 2 minutes/Cooking time – 20 minutes

juice and zest of 1 orange
1 tsp coriander seeds, crushed with a pestle and mortar
4 fresh salmon fillets
1 tbsp olive oil, plus a little extra to brush the salmon
salt and freshly ground black pepper
2 knobs of butter
1 onion, peeled and finely sliced
1 bay leaf
300g arborio risotto rice
200ml white wine
1 1/5 litres hot stock, vegetable, chicken or fish
large pinch of saffron, soaked in a little hot water
pinch of ground cinnamon (optional)
30g parmesan cheese, grated

1. Preheat the oven to 200°C/gas mark 6.
2. Put the orange juice and zest and the coriander in a small roasting dish.

3. Season the salmon with plenty of salt and pepper and brush with a little olive oil.
4. Heat a frying pan and, when it is really hot, lay the salmon fillets skin side down on the pan to sear them.
5. After a few minutes, when the skin has become crisp (it will come away from the pan easily), remove the salmon fillets from the pan and place them in the roasting dish, skin side up.
6. In a non-stick saucepan, sauté the onion with the bay leaf very slowly in a generous knob of butter and a tablespoon of oil until it becomes translucent. Heat up the stock in another pan.
7. Add the rice to the onion and stir it around so that it is well coated with the oil.
8. Add the wine and stir constantly until it is absorbed. Add a ladleful of stock and stir until it is absorbed into the rice. Add the saffron and then keep adding the stock, stirring all the time. Let the rice absorb the stock before you add the next ladleful.
9. Pop the salmon in the oven – it should take about 10 minutes to cook, but it can rest if the risotto is not ready.
10. The risotto should take about 15 minutes to cook. When the rice is almost cooked (al dente) but there is still a bit of liquid in the pan which has not yet been absorbed, add the grated parmesan, the cinnamon and a large knob of butter. Stir and leave for a couple of minutes.
11. Take the salmon out of the oven. Place the fillets on 4 warmed plates. Reduce the juice a little by boiling it for a couple of minutes on the hob. Serve the risotto with the salmon and pour over the lovely orangey juices. Fresh green beans complement this dish very well.

Saffron Rice

A tasty and exotic alternative to plain basmati rice; medium G.I and good for endurance.

Saffron rice is really easy to make and so much tastier than plain rice. It is good with kebabs, salmon steaks or any other oily fish, tagines and casseroles. It could also be a meal in itself with a nice green salad. Basmati rice is a great fuel for athletes, it is low in fat and an excellent source of vitamin E, B vitamins (thiamin and niacin) and potassium. It has a medium G.I. so will break down fairly gradually, and it is easy to digest. The almonds are full of magnesium and potassium and the cranberries are a good antioxidant and brimming with vitamin C. If you use brown basmati you will need to cook it for a bit longer and add a little more water.

Nutrition per serving

Energy (kcal)	526	Protein (g)	8
Carbohydrate (g)	60	Fat (g)	29
Of which sugars (g)	7	Of which saturates (g)	15
Salt (g)	0.9	Fibre (g)	1.5

Serves 4

Prep time – 5 minutes/Cooking time – 10–15 minutes

100g unsalted butter
1 cinnamon stick
6 cardamom pods, bruised with a pestle and mortar
1 bay leaf
4 crushed back peppercorns
250g white basmati rice, rinsed until the water runs clear and drained
50g flaked almonds (pistachios are also nice as an alternative)
75g dried cranberries (find them with the sultanas and raisins in the supermarket)
pinch of saffron, soaked in a few tbsp boiling water and left to infuse for 10 minutes

salt
freshly chopped parsley or coriander to decorate

1. Melt the butter in a large saucepan and then add the cinnamon stick, cardamom, bay leaf and black peppercorns. Gently sauté over a low heat for a few minutes until you can smell the aroma of the spices.
2. Add the rice and stir to coat with the butter.
3. Add the nuts, cranberries and the saffron water and then pour over enough water to cover the rice by about 1cm. Add some salt at this stage. Bring to the boil, cover tightly and simmer gently for 10 minutes, or until the rice is cooked. The rice will soak up the water, so you will not have to drain it.
4. Fluff up with a fork and serve in a dish, sprinkled with the fresh herbs.

Spicy Chicken and Chickpea Pilaf with Yoghurt and Cucumber Sauce

Low-fat, low-G.I. meal – good 'endurance' food for carbo-loading before a race.

It is important to follow three golden rules when cooking a pilaf – firstly, cook everything slowly on a gentle heat; secondly, use really good-quality basmati rice; and thirdly, let the pilaf stand for a while before you serve it. If you follow these rules, your end result will be light and fluffy and really flavoursome. This pilaf is a nicely balanced, low-fat meal, providing plenty of low-G.I., slow-burning carbohydrate with the basmati rice and the chickpeas, good protein from the chicken and too many vitamins and minerals to list from the herbs and spices; absolutely fantastic for training and really tasty and easy to cook too.

Nutrition per serving

Energy (kcal)	608	Protein (g)	28
Carbohydrate (g)	99	Fat (g)	13.5
Of which sugars (g)	17	Of which saturates (g)	3
Salt (g)	0.9	Fibre (g)	6.5

Serves 4
Prep time – 5 minutes/Cooking time – 20 minutes

For the pilaf

2 tbsp oil – groundnut or sunflower
1 tbsp garam masala, pounded with a pestle and mortar (or crush a mix of 6 cardamom pods, 8 cloves, 1 tsp coriander seeds, ½ tsp allspice and ½ tsp cumin seeds)
1 tsp turmeric
2 cinnamon sticks
2 onions, peeled and sliced finely
1 clove of garlic, peeled and crushed
2 bay leaves
4 skinless and boneless chicken thighs, cut into chunks

2 tomatoes, chopped
handful of sultanas (optional)
1 green chilli, deseeded and chopped
300g basmati rice, rinsed a couple of times, soaked for 30 minutes and then drained
450ml chicken stock
1 x 400g can chickpeas, drained
squeeze of lemon
fresh coriander or mint, coarsely chopped, to decorate
handful of cashew nuts, lightly toasted in the oven
2cm piece of fresh ginger, peeled and grated

For the yoghurt and cucumber sauce
½ tsp cumin
½ tsp ground coriander
¼ tsp chilli powder
½ small cucumber, chopped
handful of chopped fresh mint
250g low-fat natural yoghurt

1. Heat 2 tablespoons of oil into a large pan with a tight-fitting lid and gently fry the pilaf spices for a minute, stirring all the time so that they don't burn. Add the onion, garlic and bay leaves and sauté gently for about 5 minutes until the onion starts to soften and become brown, then add the chicken and stir it around for a minute or two to seal it.
2. Add the tomatoes, the sultanas and the green chilli and cook, stirring all the time, for another few minutes.
3. Add the rice, gently turning it around in the onion mixture for a minute to coat it, and then add the stock. (If you are using home-made stock you may need to taste it before you add it to check that it is salty enough; if you are using shop-bought stock, it will have enough salt already). There should be enough liquid to just cover the rice.
4. Bring the stock to the boil, stir, then cover and simmer at a really low heat for 10 minutes or until the rice is almost cooked.

Meanwhile mix together the yoghurt sauce ingredients and set aside.

5. Stir the chickpeas into the chicken and rice and cook for a couple of minutes. Check for seasoning, add a squeeze of lemon and sprinkle with chopped coriander or mint and the cashew nuts.
6. Leave to rest, covered, for a couple of minutes before serving.
7. Serve with yoghurt sauce, mango chutney and warm naan or pitta bread.

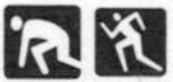

Lemon and Fennel Pilaf with Garlic Prawns

Low-G.I. energy food, light on the stomach so good for the night before a race.

I would really recommend keeping packets of frozen prawns in the freezer – a packet of good-quality peeled prawns and a packet of unpeeled tiger prawns, uncooked if possible. They are quick to defrost and are great for adding a bit of protein, omega-3 fatty acids, copper, magnesium, zinc and iron to a meal which is based mostly on carbohydrate. The pilaf is light and subtle, a perfect combination with the prawns, yet substantial enough to sustain you because it uses lower-G.I. basmati rice.

Nutrition per serving

Energy (kcal)	408	Protein (g)	12
Carbohydrate (g)	69	Fat (g)	9
Of which sugars (g)	3	Of which saturates (g)	1.5
Salt (g)	1.6	Fibre (g)	1.5

Serves 4
Prep time – 5 mins/Cooking time – 15 mins

For the pilaf
500ml fish or vegetable stock
large knob of butter or 1 tbsp oil
1 onion, peeled and finely sliced
1 small fennel bulb, finely sliced (save any green fronds for the prawns)
1 clove of garlic, peeled and crushed
1 tsp fennel seeds (find them on the spice rack in the supermarket)
300g basmati rice, rinsed and then soaked in water for 30 minutes
zest of 1 lemon
salt

For the prawns
knob of butter or 1 tbsp olive oil
12 large uncooked unpeeled prawns

1 clove of garlic, finely sliced
handful of fennel fronds or dill
juice and zest of 1 lemon
120ml white wine or Pernod

1. To make the pilaf, bring the stock to the boil in a saucepan and keep hot.
2. Heat the butter or oil in a heavy-based saucepan, then add the onion and fennel and sauté gently for a few minutes.
3. Add the garlic and the fennel seeds and sauté gently for another couple of minutes, until the onion and fennel are soft.
4. Drain the soaked rice and add it to the pan. Stir it gently so that the rice is coated with the butter and then add the stock. Taste for seasoning and add salt if necessary.
5. Bring to the boil and then simmer for 10 minutes with the pan covered with a circle of greaseproof paper and a tight-fitting lid. You can scrunch up a piece of greaseproof paper and soak it under the tap – then unscrunch it and place it over the rice mixture.
6. Remove the greaseproof paper and then check that the rice is cooked. Turn off the heat, stir in the lemon zest and leave the rice for a few minutes to rest while you sauté the prawns.
7. Heat the knob of butter or oil in a frying pan and, when hot, add the prawns.
8. Sauté on a high flame for a couple of minutes until the prawns have turned pink and are cooked through.
9. Add the garlic and the fennel fronds, the lemon juice and zest and a splash of water, white wine or Pernod and serve with the pilaf.

Thai Green Fish Curry with Rice Noodles

Great fast food – balanced, healthy and good for endurance training.

This is a regular in our household. It is healthy, good energy food, quick and easy to make and adored by everyone. Most rice noodles have a low G.I. factor and all you have to do is soak them in boiling water for a few minutes. This curry is equally good with strips of chicken thigh or breast, beef or meaty vegetables like aubergines. You can buy most ingredients for Thai curries in the supermarket these days – palm sugar and fresh kaffir lime leaves are sometimes a little elusive, so I have suggested alternatives for these.

Nutrition per serving

Energy (kcal)	583	Protein (g)	37
Carbohydrate (g)	62	Fat (g)	22
Of which sugars (g)	16	Of which saturates (g)	7
Salt (g)	1.4	Fibre (g)	4

Serves 4
Prep time – 5 minutes/Cooking time – 10–15 minutes

2 x 400ml tin of coconut milk (I use low-fat coconut milk for this recipe as it is not so thick)
4 tbsp Thai green curry paste
2cm fresh ginger, peeled and finely sliced
1 tbsp Thai fish sauce
1 tbsp palm sugar or brown sugar
8 kaffir lime leaves, 4 finely sliced, 4 whole, or the grated zest of 1 lime
500g good firm fresh fish, like monkfish, cubed, or large uncooked prawns
juice of ½ – 1 lime
bunch of fresh coriander leaves, roughly chopped
2 green chillies, deseeded and sliced lengthways
250g rice noodles

1. Heat ½ tin of coconut milk in a wok, or large pan, over a medium heat. Stir in the curry paste and the ginger and simmer gently for 2–3 minutes, stirring all the time.
2. Add the remaining coconut milk, the fish sauce, palm sugar and 4 whole lime leaves and simmer for a further 5 minutes.
3. Meanwhile prepare the rice noodles according to the instructions on the pack.
4. Add the fish to the wok and simmer for 5 minutes or until the fish is cooked. If you overcook it, it will go rubbery, so keep alert. Add the juice of ½ lime and check for seasoning, adding more fish sauce, lime juice or sugar if needed.
5. Add the noodles to the pot (you can serve them separately, if you want).
6. Sprinkle the coriander, the green chillies and the finely sliced lime leaves on top.

Red Curry Duck with Lychees and Fragrant Jasmine Rice

Great for recovery or a rest day. The rice is high G.I. and the curry is packed with nutrients.

This is one of the easiest and quickest curries you can make, especially if you use shop-bought red curry paste. I once used tinned lychees as there were no fresh ones available ... that was a mistake as they were too soft and rather tasteless – if you can't find fresh lychees use red or green grapes instead. Thai fragrant jasmine rice is a short grain white rice which is widely available. It has a high G.I. and so is perfect for replenishing your tired muscles after a heavy workout.

Nutrition per serving

Energy (kcal)	830	Protein (g)	48
Carbohydrate (g)	71	Fat (g)	41
Of which sugars (g)	15	Of which saturates (g)	25
Salt (g)	1.3	Fibre (g)	1

Serves 4
Prep time – 5 minutes/Cooking time – 50 minutes

4 duck legs
salt
2 tbsp red curry paste (use less if you like it mild)
200ml coconut cream
100ml chicken stock
1 desertspoon Thai fish sauce
1 desertspoon sugar
4 kaffir lime leaves (optional)
250g fragrant jasmine rice
16 lychees, peeled and deseeded, or seedless grapes
small handful basil or coriander leaves, chopped

1. Preheat the oven to 180°C/gas mark 4.
2. Remove the excess fat and any extra skin hanging off the sides of

the duck legs with kitchen scissors and pat dry. Sprinkle all over with a little salt and then very gently fry in a large wok or frying pan, skin side down, for about 35 minutes, until the skin becomes nice and crispy. Spoon off excess fat every now and then.

3. Spoon off any excess fat again and turn the legs over. Cook the legs for a further 10–15 minutes and then pop them onto a roasting pan, skin side up, and put them in the oven for 10–15 minutes, while you make the sauce and cook the rice.
4. Using the same frying pan that you cooked the duck in, fry the red curry paste with a tablespoon or two of coconut cream, stirring all the time for 2 minutes, then add the remaining coconut cream, chicken stock, fish sauce, sugar and the lime leaves.
5. Prepare the jasmine rice. Rinse the rice in cold water and then place in a pan with 600ml water (enough to cover the rice by ½ inch, or to the first joint of your middle finger). Cover with a tight-fitting lid, bring to the boil and simmer for 7–10 minutes, or until all the water has been absorbed. Turn off the heat and leave for 4–5 minutes. Uncover the pan and fluff up the rice to serve. It is authentic not to use salted water – the rice is a completely plain accompaniment to the curry.
6. Put the duck legs back in the pan to finish cooking in the sauce, crispy skin side up. Simmer for a few minutes and then add the lychees and the basil or coriander.
7. Taste for seasoning. You may need to add a little extra stock or some lime juice if the sauce is too rich and thick.
8. Serve with steamed jasmine rice to soak up the juices.

Thai Sweet Basil Chicken with Rice Noodles

A delicious way to carbo-load if you are preparing for a race.

Thai sweet basil has a distinctive taste, similar to European sweet basil, but with a much more pronounced aniseed flavour. You can buy it in most oriental supermarkets, and it is an excellent source of vitamin K, A and C plus minerals such as iron, calcium, magnesium and manganese. If you cannot get hold of Thai sweet basil then just use the standard European variety – not quite as authentic, but delicious all the same. This meal is great because it is packed with goodness and is very versatile – fine for midweek, but good enough for a dinner party. It is fresh and healthy, and provides a really good balance of carbohydrate, protein, vitamins and minerals. I prefer to use free-range organic chicken thighs for this dish – the meat is darker, juicier and contains more iron – but any chicken will do.

Nutrition per serving

Energy (kcal)	635	Protein (g)	34
Carbohydrate (g)	54	Fat (g)	33
Of which sugars (g)	7	Of which saturates (g)	6
Salt (g)	2.6	Fibre (g)	5

Serves 4
Prep time – 5 minutes/Cooking time – 15 minutes

4 tbsp groundnut or sunflower oil
2 small fresh red chillies, deseeded and chopped (add the seeds, plus some whole chillies, if you want more heat)
8–10cm piece (45g) fresh ginger, peeled and cut into very thin strips
4 cloves of garlic, peeled and crushed
8 skinless, boneless chicken thigh fillets or 4 chicken breasts (organic free range if possible)
2 tsp sugar (palm sugar if you have some)
100g chopped peanuts or cashew nuts, or 2 tbsp satay sauce
3–4 tbsp Thai fish sauce

2 large handfuls green beans, cut into half
2 tbsp oyster sauce
10 tbsp fresh (a very large bunch) Thai basil leaves (use regular basil if you cannot find any)
250g plain rice noodles, cooked according to pack instructions
a few basil leaves and lime wedges to serve

1. Heat the oil in a frying pan or wok. Add the chilli, ginger and garlic and fry for 20–30 seconds.
2. Add the chicken and stir-fry for a minute or so until sealed.
3. Stir in the sugar, chopped nuts or satay sauce and 3 tsbp fish sauce and then fry gently for about 10 minutes or until the meat is cooked. Add a little water or stock if it looks a bit dry.
4. While the chicken is cooking, prepare the noodles according to pack instructions.
5. Add the green beans to the chicken and continue to stir-fry for a 2–3 minutes.
6. Stir in the oyster sauce and then add the basil leaves. Taste for seasoning – you may need more chilli, fish sauce or sugar.
7. Serve with the noodles, garnished with basil leaves and a wedge of lime.

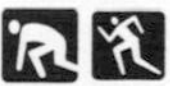

Beef Massaman Curry with Butternut Squash and Potato

Nutritious dish for your training diet – the protein in the beef and the peanuts helps to build and repair muscles, the basil contains calcium and vitamin K to help your bones and the spices help reduce inflammation and muscle spasms.

Massaman curry is a Thai dish with Indian influences, usually made with beef or chicken. It consists of a mixture of Thai ingredients such as coconut milk, roasted peanuts, fish sauce, tamarind and palm sugar, plus Indian spices such as cinnamon, cardamom and bay. It generally has less heat than a traditional red or green curry and my version with potatoes, butternut squash and basil makes a very warming and substantial meal. I sometimes serve this as a soup with some chillies and peanuts sprinkled on top, in which case I add a little more coconut milk to thin the sauce. Otherwise it is good with some plain boiled brown basmati rice, which, combined with the potato and butternut squash, makes for a really good endurance meal.

Nutrition per serving

Energy (kcal)	660	Protein (g)	30
Carbohydrate (g)	99	Fat (g)	19
Of which sugars (g)	13	Of which saturates (g)	6
Salt (g)	0.9	Fibre (g)	3.5

Serves 4

Prep time – 5 minutes/Cooking time – 1 hour

400ml coconut milk
3 tbsp massaman curry paste (jars are available in most supermarkets and Asian stores)
3 cardamom pods, bruised gently with a pestle and mortar
1 cinnamon stick
2 bay leaves
300g lean stewing steak, cut into 1cm strips

30g roasted peanuts, plus some extra to serve
1 onion, peeled and quartered, or handful of small baby onions, peeled and left whole
1 large waxy potato, peeled and cut into 1cm chunks
250g butternut squash, peeled and cut into 1cm chunks
300g brown or white basmati rice
1 tbsp fish sauce
1 tsp palm sugar or brown sugar
squeeze of lime juice
handful of basil leaves torn roughly, plus a few chopped basil leaves to serve
1 fresh red chilli, deseeded and finely sliced

1. In a large frying pan or wok, heat up 60ml coconut milk. When it is boiling, mix in the massaman curry paste and stir to combine. Cook for a minute at a high heat and then add the beef. Stir to coat the beef all over with the paste and cook for a few minutes, stirring all the time to seal the beef.
2. Add another 200ml coconut milk, 100ml water, the cardamom, cinnamon stick and bay leaves and bring to the boil. Turn the heat down to a simmer and cook on a low heat, uncovered, for about 20 minutes.
3. Add the peanuts, onion, potato and butternut squash and the rest of the coconut milk and continue to simmer for another 30 minutes until the vegetables are just tender.
4. Meanwhile cook the rice according to the pack instructions.
5. When the meat and vegetables are tender and the sauce has thickened up, add the fish sauce, sugar, lime juice and test for seasoning. If it needs more salt, add a little more fish sauce. Likewise, if you think it could be sweeter, add some more sugar. Add the basil leaves.
6. Serve with extra peanuts, chopped basil and sliced red chillies to sprinkle over.

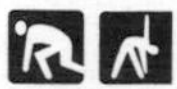

Penang Prawn Curry with Fragrant Steamed Jasmine Rice

Good to eat to help muscles recover after a big workout – the jasmine rice has a high G.I. and the curry is full of nutrients to help your bones, replace lost salts and reduce muscle inflammation.

Thai curries are quick, easy, healthy and really delicious. The trick to a Thai curry is to create the perfect harmony of heat, salt, sweet and sour by using a basic mix of coconut milk, fish sauce, curry paste, chilli, lime and sugar. You can make your own curry paste if you have the time and the inclination, but really good ready-made pastes are available in the shops now. If you have an Asian store nearby, you will find the ingredients will be cheaper and very authentic, but you should find everything you need in your local supermarket too. This curry is absolutely crammed with nutrition – peanuts, prawns, green and red vegetables and basil. What's more, the aromas are so tempting, you'll want to eat it straight away.

Nutrition per serving

Energy (kcal)	785	Protein (g)	50
Carbohydrate (g)	92	Fat (g)	27
Of which sugars (g)	30	Of which saturates (g)	9
Salt (g)	6	Fibre (g)	4

Serves 4
Prep time – 5 minutes (add another 5 if you make your own curry paste)/Cooking time – 15 minutes

For the curry and rice

4 tbsp Penang curry paste (see below), or use red curry paste as an alternative
250g Thai jasmine rice
1 litre coconut milk
4–6 tbsp fish sauce

2 tbsp palm sugar or brown sugar
2 tbsp unsalted peanuts, ground in the blender, or use chunky peanut butter
4 handfuls sugar snap peas
500g uncooked, peeled prawns
2 red peppers, deseeded and cut into strips
12 kaffir lime leaves, torn into strips
juice of ½ a lime
4 fresh red chillies, deseeded and cut into strips
2 large handfuls Thai basil leaves (use regular basil if you cannot get hold of Thai basil)

For the Penang curry paste

4 dried chillies
1 tsp coriander seeds
1 tsp cumin seeds
½ tsp black peppercorns
3 shallots, peeled
2 cloves of garlic, peeled
2 stalks of lemongrass
1cm piece fresh ginger or galangal, peeled
4 tbsp fresh coriander root
4 kaffir lime leaves
½ tsp dried shrimp paste
1 tbsp peanuts
2 tbsp water

For the nam pla prik

3 large chillies, including seeds, finely sliced
1 clove garlic, finely sliced
100ml fish sauce
juice of ½ a lime

1. To make your own curry paste, dry fry the chillies, coriander seeds, cumin seeds and black peppercorns in a pan for 3 minutes,

until you can smell the fragrant aroma of the spices. Then pop into blender with the remaining curry paste ingredients and whiz until smooth. (Quantities do not have to be too exact).

2. Combine all the ingredients for the nam pla prik and pour into a small serving bowl.
3. Prepare the jasmine rice. Rinse in cold water and then place in a pan with 600ml water (enough to cover the rice by ½ inch, or to the first joint of your middle finger). Cover with a tight-fitting lid, bring to the boil and simmer for 7–10 minutes, or until all the water has been absorbed. Turn off the heat and leave for 4–5 minutes. Uncover the pan and fluff up the rice to serve. It is authentic not to use salted water – the rice is a completely plain accompaniment to the curry.
4. Heat half the coconut milk in a wok or large frying pan, bring to the boil then add 2 tbsp of the curry paste. Simmer for 2–3 minutes, stirring all the time.
5. Add 4 tbsp fish sauce and the palm sugar and stir, then add the peanuts and the rest of the coconut milk and simmer for a minute or two.
6. Add the peas, prawns, red pepper, the kaffir lime leaves, lime juice and 2 chillies and simmer for a few minutes until the prawns are pink and the vegetables are just cooked.
7. Taste for seasoning – add more chilli if you need more heat, or perhaps more fish sauce, some lime juice or sugar – try to get a balance that suits your taste.
8. Transfer to a serving bowl and sprinkle with the basil leaves and the remaining chilli.
9. Serve with the rice and the nam pla prik.

polenta and gnocchi

'I crave savoury foods post race due to all the sugary supplements, gels and drinks.' Llewellyn Holmes, personal trainer, triathlete and road/mountainbike racer. World Xterra Championships (British age group winner and 2nd place) and Ironman (3rd place).

Fresh Gnocchi

Great for a delicious and filling post-workout meal.

Fresh home-made gnocchi is lighter than the shop-bought version. It is much less trouble to make than you might think, and you can make it in advance and store it in the freezer. Gnocchi is good with pesto, with creamy sauces such as the mushroom sauce in the next recipe, or with fresh herbs, olive oil and parmesan. The recipe is for eight servings so that you can make some and freeze the rest. It only takes a few minutes to cook and so is perfect to eat when you are really tired after a big training session.

Nutrition per serving

Energy (kcal)	247	Protein (g)	8
Carbohydrate (g)	47	Fat (g)	4
Of which sugars (g)	1.5	Of which saturates (g)	0.5
Salt (g)	0.8	Fibre (g)	2

Serves 8
Prep time - 30 minutes/Cooking time - 3 minutes

1kg floury potatoes (King Edward are good)
1 egg, lightly beaten
300g plain flour
1 tsp salt
freshly ground black pepper
olive oil to serve

1. Boil the potatoes in their skins in salted water for about 25 minutes or until tender.
2. Remove the potatoes and, when they are cool enough to handle, carefully peel them with a sharp knife.
3. Mash or grate the potatoes, or mince them in a potato ricer if you have one.
4. Add the egg and mix in thoroughly, then mix the flour, salt and plenty of black pepper. Use your hands to bring the mixture together into a dough.
5. Put the dough on a floured surface and gently knead it. Then take a handful of the dough and roll it into a sausage shape. Using a sharp knife, cut into little gnocchi (oval balls), about 1½–2cm long and put them into a floured container. They are now ready to cook.
6. Bring a large saucepan of salted water to the boil. You need to cook the gnocchi in batches, about a handful at a time, so they don't crowd the pan. Plunge each batch unto the boiling water for about 2 minutes until they rise to the surface. Remove them with a slotted spoon and serve immediately with your favourite sauce or drizzled with olive oil and plenty of black pepper.

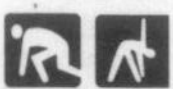

Gnocchi with Mushroom Sauce

Simple and nutritious medium- to high-G.I. carbohydrate meal for recovery.

Gnocchi has a medium G.I. of 68 and the mushroom sauce is very soothing. It is really simple to prepare so is great to eat after a big run when you are tired. There is something about this meal that makes you sleep very well!

Nutrition per serving

Energy (kcal)	566	Protein (g)	11
Carbohydrate (g)	64	Fat (g)	29
Of which sugars (g)	5	Of which saturates (g)	16
Salt (g)	1	Fibre (g)	4

Serves 2–3
Prep time – 5 minutes/Cooking time – 5–10 minutes

500g fresh gnocchi (see page 174)
1 tbsp olive oil
1 small, mild onion, peeled and finely chopped
1 bay leaf (optional)
250g chestnut mushrooms, finely sliced
1 clove of garlic, peeled and crushed
salt and freshly ground black pepper
splash of white wine
300ml crème fraîche
1 tsp wholegrain mustard
handful of flat-leaved parsley or tarragon chopped, plus some extra to sprinkle on top

1. In a large frying pan with a lid, sauté the onion with the bay leaf very, very gently in the oil for 5–10 minutes, until soft.
2. Add the mushrooms, the garlic and a pinch of salt, cover and sweat on a very low heat for another 5 minutes or so.

3. Take the lid off, turn up the heat, add the wine and reduce for a few minutes.
4. Add the crème fraîche, the mustard and herbs and cook for another minute or so. Season with salt and freshly ground black pepper. Remove the bay leaf.
5. Meanwhile, cook the gnocchi, according to pack instructions if using shop-bought, drain, then spoon into the mushroom mixture and serve in some nice big pasta bowls.
6. Decorate with some more fresh herbs. This dish goes well with a fresh rocket salad sprinkled with pine nuts.

Soft Polenta with Wild Mushroom Ragu

Great for training, with a good balance of protein, minerals and low- to medium-G.I. carbohydrate

This is a delicious and comforting dish, quick and easy to make and great for training. The polenta is medium G.I. and the mushrooms have a low G.I of 40, so all in all this will give you a good level of endurance. My son finds it very difficult to eat lunch before his school rugby matches as he takes them very seriously and gets extremely nervous. I find that he manages to stomach this polenta dish as it is easy to eat, yet filling and sustaining. I tend to cook my polenta with stock or water, as I find milk is too heavy, especially if I am exercising afterwards.

Nutrition per serving

Energy (kcal)	320	Protein (g)	9
Carbohydrate (g)	38	Fat (g)	14.5
Of which sugars (g)	3.5	Of which saturates (g)	3.5
Salt (g)	0.7	Fibre (g)	3.5

Serves 4

Prep time – 5–10 minutes + soaking time for the dried mushrooms/Cooking time – 10–15 minutes (a little longer if using slow-cook polenta)

400g polenta (instant or slow-cook)
2 tbsp olive oil
2 shallots, peeled and finely sliced
1 clove of garlic, peeled and finely sliced
250g mushrooms, sliced (best to use a mixture of fresh field and chestnut mushrooms and a 25g pack of dried wild mushrooms such as porcini, soaked for 30 minutes)
handful of fresh mint, thyme or flat-leaved parsley, chopped
splash of dry white wine or sherry (optional)
200g cherry tomatoes, halved
splash of balsamic vinegar

2–3 tbsp fruity extra virgin olive oil
salt and freshly ground black pepper
grated parmesan cheese to serve

1. Cook the polenta according to pack instructions for soft polenta. You can cook it with water or stock, or even a mixture or stock and milk, whatever you prefer. As with all polenta recipes, use a large pan as the mixture will spit out at you. The polenta should be the consistency of semolina, or porridge.
2. Gently sauté the shallots and garlic in the olive oil until the shallot is soft and translucent.
3. Turn up the heat and add the mushrooms. Cook for about 5 minutes and then add the fresh herbs (save some for decoration), wine and the tomatoes.
4. Cook for a further 5 minutes, until the tomatoes have softened.
5. Add a splash of balsamic vinegar.
6. Add a good glug of extra virgin olive oil and some salt and pepper to the polenta and spoon onto individual plates.
7. Spoon the mushroom mix on top of the polenta, drizzle with more extra virgin olive oil, an extra sprinkling of fresh herbs and some parmesan shavings and serve immediately. It works well accompanied with a crisp, green salad

Venetian Polenta with Baby Shrimps

Great for training, with a good balance of protein, minerals and medium-G.I. carbohydrate. Also makes a good dinner party starter.

This is based on a dish I was lucky enough to come across on a visit to Venice – *schie con polenta*, a delicious dish of baby shrimps from the Venice lagoon, sautéed with garlic and parsley and served on a bed of soft polenta. We cannot get hold of these little shrimps in the UK very easily, so my version of the dish uses any type of small shrimps that I can get hold of. My fishmonger supplies vacuum packs of tiny brown shrimps which are cheap and perfect for this dish. Otherwise, just use a pack of peeled frozen shrimps from the supermarket – the smallest ones you can find.

Nutrition per serving

Energy (kcal)	300	Protein (g)	21
Carbohydrate (g)	34	Fat (g)	7
Of which sugars (g)	2	Of which saturates (g)	1
Salt (g)	1.6	Fibre (g)	1.5

Serves 4
Prep time – 1 minute/Cooking time – 5 minutes (longer if using slow-cook polenta)

2 tbsp olive oil
2 cloves of garlic, peeled and sliced finely
2 tsp fresh rosemary, chopped
400g peeled baby shrimps
splash of dry white wine
400g polenta (instant or slow-cook)
extra virgin olive oil
salt and freshly ground black pepper

1. Gently sauté the garlic and the rosemary in the olive oil for a minute or two.

2. Add the shrimps and a splash of wine and warm through – if you are using uncooked shrimps, cook them until they turn pink.
3. Cook the polenta according to pack instructions for soft polenta. Remember to use a large pan and a long spoon as the polenta will spit out at you. The polenta should be the consistency of semolina, or porridge.
4. Add a good glug of olive oil and some salt and pepper to the polenta and spoon onto individual plates.
5. Spoon the shrimp, garlic and rosemary mix on top of the polenta, drizzle with more olive oil and serve immediately.
6. Accompany with a crisp, green salad.

couscous

'I find couscous with chickpeas a wonderful pre-training carbohydrate – full of nutrition and filling, but light and easy to digest.' Martin Picton, Crown Court Judge, marathon runner. Best event – Berlin Marathon 2007.

'Your chicken, preserved lemon and green olives tagine with that delicious couscous hit the spot perfectly after the Bristol Half.' Kate Persad, Practice Manager, mother and half-marathon runner. Best event – Bristol Half Marathon 2008.

Algerian Chicken Tagine with Apricots

Ideal for a Saturday night before a big Sunday morning training session or for an informal dinner party.

I adore North African tagines. Best eaten with plain couscous, they are easy to cook, temptingly aromatic and they make the kitchen smell gorgeous. A tagine pot is nice to have but not a necessity – any good heavy-bottomed casserole dish will do. Hot and sultry summer's evening or chilly autumn night, this dish is equally appealing, conjuring up dreams of exotic holidays. The combination of chicken with apricots and fresh coriander provides a good balance of protein, fibre, vitamins and minerals and the addition of the couscous balances the meal perfectly. Spanish smoked paprika, orange flower water and ras-el-hanout are now widely available in supermarkets and are definitely worth adding to your store cupboard as they can add real authenticity to any Spanish or North-African dish.

Nutrition per serving

Energy (kcal)	673	Protein (g)	53
Carbohydrate (g)	76	Fat (g)	20
Of which sugars (g)	17	Of which saturates (g)	5
Salt (g)	2.5	Fibre (g)	6

Serves 4
Prep time – 5 minutes/Cooking time – 40 minutes

For the tagine

8 free-range chicken thighs or 4 chicken quarters, on the bone
2 tbsp flour, seasoned with pinch of salt, pepper and paprika
2 tbsp sunflower oil
2 onions, peeled and chopped
2 bay leaves (optional)
4 cloves of garlic, peeled and finely chopped
5cm piece of fresh ginger, peeled and grated
1 tsp paprika (or better still, Spanish smoked paprika)
4 tsp ras-el-hanout spice mix (use Moroccan spice mix as an alternative)
1 cinnamon stick
1 pinch of saffron, soaked in a little boiling water for 10 minutes
chicken stock to cover
large handful of ready-soaked, dried apricots, halved
2 tsp honey
splash of orange flower water (or use zest of ½ an orange as an alternative)
large handful of fresh coriander leaves, roughly chopped

For the couscous

250g couscous (wholemeal if you can get it)
1 tsp salt
knob of butter
handful of flaked almonds, roasted in the oven at 180°C/gas mark 4 for 5 minutes

1. Coat the chicken in the flour. Heat the oil in a heavy-bottomed casserole dish and brown the chicken gently for about 5 minutes.
2. Remove the chicken and then gently sauté the onion with the bay leaf until soft.
3. Add the garlic, ginger and the spices (except the saffron) and sauté for a couple of minutes until you smell a delicious aroma being released.
4. Add the chicken, the saffron and enough stock to cover the chicken. Bring to the boil, cover and put in the oven for about 30–40 minutes, or until the chicken is cooked. Halfway through the cooking, add the apricots.
5. Prepare the couscous – rinse in cold water and then place in a bowl with the salt and the butter. Pour over 300ml boiling water and leave for 5 minutes (check pack for exact quantity of water and how long to leave it). Fluff up the couscous gently with a fork, adding the almonds as you do so.
6. When the chicken is cooked, add the honey and the orange flower water and return to the oven for a few more minutes. Boil down the juice (on the hob) if too thin, spoon off any excess fat and then add the fresh coriander.
7. Taste for seasoning. You may want to add more salt and pepper or spice, maybe even a squeeze of lemon.
8. Serve with the couscous and a fresh rocket salad.

Chicken Tagine with Couscous, Green Olives and Preserved Lemons

Delicious, balanced meal, good fuel for endurance training.

This is a very warming, exotic and comforting dish. The couscous is low to medium G.I., and the tagine is low fat and packed with vitamins. I served this on the night England lost the Rugby World Cup Final. I prepared it in advance, soaked the couscous at half time, and we ate it after the match. It seemed to cheer our party somewhat and I must say that I was nicely fuelled for my run along the rather hilly Devon coastal path the following morning. Preserved lemons are basically lemons that have been preserved in brine. They are used a lot in Mediterranean and North African cooking and are widely available here in the UK now.

Nutrition per serving

Energy (kcal)	505	Protein (g)	29
Carbohydrate (g)	61	Fat (g)	18
Of which sugars (g)	7	Of which saturates (g)	3
Salt (g)	4	Fibre (g)	4

Serves 4
Prep time – 5 minutes + marinating time/
Cooking time – 40–50 minutes

For the marinade

3 tbsp good olive oil
¼ tsp cayenne pepper
¼ tsp black pepper
½ tsp ground turmeric
1 tsp ground cumin
1 tsp ground coriander
1 tsp sweet paprika
1 tsp ground ginger
1 tsp salt
3 cloves garlic, peeled and crushed
3 tbsp water

For the tagine

8 skinless free-range chicken thighs, each cut into about three pieces
2 tbsp olive oil
2 large onions, peeled and finely sliced
flour for coating the chicken
1 cinnamon stick
big bunch of flat-leaf parsley, chopped (keep some aside to sprinkle on top)
big bunch of coriander leaves, chopped (keep some aside to sprinkle on top)
chicken stock to cover
2 preserved lemons (plus 1 tbsp of the juice from the jar)
about 20 nice green olives (pitted if you wish)
¼ tsp smoked paprika

For the couscous

250g couscous (wholemeal if you can get it)
1 tsp salt
1 tbsp olive oil

1. Mix together the marinade ingredients and combine the chicken. Leave in the fridge overnight or for as long as you can. Bring the chicken back to room temperature.
2. Heat a couple of tablespoons of olive oil in a tagine or heavy-bottomed casserole dish, add the onions and cook gently for about 10 minutes. Remove the onions and set them aside.
3. Remove the chicken from the marinade and lightly coat with flour (just put some flour into a plastic bag with the chicken and shake it about a little). Increase the heat under the casserole, add some more oil and then brown the chicken quickly. Keep the marinade aside.
4. Pop the onions back into the pot and add the reserved marinade, the cinnamon stick, the chopped herbs and enough chicken stock to cover the chicken. Cover and bring to the boil, then reduce the heat and simmer for about 30 minutes until the chicken is cooked.
5. Prepare the couscous – rinse in cold water and then place in a

bowl with the salt and the olive oil. Pour over 300ml boiling water and leave for 5 minutes (check pack for exact quantity of water and how long to leave it). Fluff up the couscous gently with a fork.

6. Slice the preserved lemons thinly and discard the pips and flesh.
7. Add the lemons, the preserved lemon juice, the olives and the smoked paprika to the simmering chicken and cook for a further 5 minutes.
8. Test for seasoning – it may need more salt and pepper, perhaps an extra kick with a sprinkle of cayenne, cumin or coriander, or some lemon juice.
9. Sprinkle with the fresh herbs you set aside and serve with plain couscous.

Couscous with Slow-cooked Lamb Shanks

A warming and substantial meal – ideal to come home to after a race.

I prepared this for my husband and a couple of his friends after they completed the 120 mile cycle ride from London to Canterbury, following the route of Stage 1 of the Tour de France. They were completely exhausted! My butcher sells his lamb shanks already marinated, which I must say makes life easier, but it is easy to do at home and it makes the house smell delicious. You can prepare it the day before; in fact the flavours are better if you do so. Try experimenting with different spice mixes, or add a can of chickpeas or butter beans for extra nutrition.

Nutrition per serving

Energy (kcal)	720	Protein (g)	49
Carbohydrate (g)	60	Fat (g)	29
Of which sugars (g)	17	Of which saturates (g)	10
Salt (g)	2.5	Fibre (g)	4.5

Serves 4
Prep time – 5 mins, plus marinating time/
Cooking time – 4 hours

For the lamb

4 lamb shanks
2cm piece of fresh ginger, peeled and grated
2 x 400g tins chopped plum tomatoes
zest and juice of 1 orange
zest and juice of 1 lemon
250ml red wine
sprig of rosemary
3 cloves of garlic, peeled and crushed
1 tsp ground cinnamon
1 tsp ground cumin
1 tsp coriander seeds, crushed

1 tsp peppercorns, crushed
¼ tsp grated nutmeg
2 tbsp olive oil
1 tbsp balsamic vinegar
salt
bunch of fresh coriander leaves

For the yoghurt sauce
250g low-fat natural yoghurt
pinch of salt
pinch of sugar
1 tsp ground cumin
pinch of chilli powder
freshly ground black pepper
handful mint leaves, finely chopped

For the couscous
250g couscous
knob of butter
1 tsp salt
3 cardamom pods, crushed
25g flaked almonds, lightly roasted

1. Mix all the ingredients for the lamb shanks (except the fresh coriander) together in a bowl and add the lamb shanks. Leave to marinate for up to 24 hours.
2. Preheat the oven to 220°C/gas mark 7.
3. Lay out four pieces of tin foil big enough to wrap up each shank (about 30cm x 30cm).
4. Place ¼ of the marinade and a lamb shank in each foil square and wrap up into a loose parcel.
5. Place the foil parcels into a casserole dish, cover, and cook in the hot oven for 20–30 minutes (until you can smell the cooking).
6. Turn down the oven to 150°C/gas mark 2 and leave for 3½ hours.
7. When ready, take the casserole dish out of the oven and carefully remove the foil. The lamb shanks should be falling off the bone and there should be plenty of delicious sauce.

8. Check for seasoning – I often add an extra clove of crushed garlic, a pinch of smoked paprika and some extra spices at this point.
9. Mix together all the ingredients for the yoghurt sauce and leave in the fridge for 30 minutes or so for the flavours to infuse.
10. To prepare the couscous, place the couscous in a bowl with the salt and the butter. Pour over 300ml of boiling water and leave for 5 minutes (check the pack for exact quantity of water and how long to leave it).
11. Meanwhile, roast the almonds for 5 minutes at 180°C/gas mark 4.
12. Remove the seeds from the cardamom pods and crush them. Fluff up the couscous gently with a fork, adding the nuts and cardamom as you do so. Check for seasoning.
13. When ready to serve, sprinkle the chopped fresh coriander over the lamb and serve with the couscous, yoghurt sauce and a green salad.

Fillet of Salmon with Green Couscous

A perfect meal for training but good enough to serve to guests as a summery lunch.

Every delicious mouthful of this meal will do you good. High in protein, low in saturated fat and cholesterol and a great source of omega-3 fatty acids, salmon is a great food to incorporate into your regular diet. The couscous is only 'green' because it is packed with healthy green vegetables and herbs. It looks enticingly fresh on the plate against the pink salmon. I am becoming a great fan of cold-pressed rapeseed oil. It has a distinct yellow colour and is a great alternative to olive oil. It is reported to be one of the most heart-friendly oils available, containing more omega-3 and less saturated fat than olive oil, plus vitamin E. It can't match the peppery, fruity flavour of olive oil for salad dressings, but it is especially good for frying. It can be heated to a high temperature without losing its flavour or its nutrients and will crisp up foods beautifully – great for cooking salmon.

Nutrition per serving

Energy (kcal)	600	Protein (g)	37
Carbohydrate (g)	50	Fat (g)	32
Of which sugars (g)	3	Of which saturates (g)	5
Salt (g)	1.5	Fibre (g)	3

Serves 4
Prep time – 2 minutes/Cooking time – 10–15 minutes

250g couscous (wholemeal if you can get it)
1 tsp salt
1 tbsp rapeseed oil (use sunflower or olive oil as an alternative)
2 courgettes, cut into thin slices with a sharp knife, lengthways
4 fresh salmon fillets (organic, wild salmon is best, but any fillets will do)
juice of ½ a lemon
2 large handfuls of fresh herbs (coriander, mint, flat-leaf parsley, dill, whatever you can get hold of), chopped

2–3 tbsp extra virgin olive oil
1 tsp ground cumin
handful of pine nuts, roasted in the oven at 180°C/gas mark 4 for 5 minutes
wedges of lemon or lime to serve

1. Preheat the oven to 170°C/gas mark 3.
2. Prepare the couscous – rinse in cold water and then place in a bowl with the salt and a tbsp of extra virgin olive oil. Pour over 300ml boiling water and leave for 5 minutes (check pack for exact quantity of water and how long to leave it). Fluff up the couscous gently with a fork.
3. Heat a pan or griddle and brush the courgette slices with a little rapeseed oil. Quickly fry the courgette for a minute or two and set aside. Brush the salmon with the rapeseed oil and season with a little salt.
4. Place the salmon skin side down on the griddle and cook on a medium heat for a few minutes. When the salmon comes away easily from the pan, turn it over and seal all over. Cook gently for another few minutes, squeeze the lemon juice over it and then transfer the salmon to an ovenproof dish and pop it into the oven for 5 minutes. The salmon is cooked when it is springy to the touch. Let it rest on a warm plate while you finish off the couscous.
5. Add the herbs and courgette to the couscous and then mix it all in with another 1–2 tbsp extra virgin olive oil, a squeeze of lemon juice and the cumin. Sprinkle the pine nuts over the top.
6. Serve the salmon with the couscous and a wedge of lemon or lime.

Griddled Tuna Steak on a Bed of Spiced Cranberry Couscous with Mango and Avocado Salsa.

Excellent balanced, healthy, low-fat meal, good for training but equally good enough for a summer supper party.

This meal just oozes flavour. It is packed with goodness and is equally good either before or after a workout. The salsa contains a wide variety of vitamins and the couscous is a good low-fat, medium-G.I. carbohydrate. It goes without saying that fresh tuna is one of the better sources of omega-3 fatty acids – good for your heart and good for your brain.

Nutrition per serving

Energy (kcal)	420	Protein (g)	27
Carbohydrate (g)	58	Fat (g)	10
Of which sugars (g)	10	Of which saturates (g)	2
Salt (g)	1.2	Fibre (g)	5

Serves 4
Prep time – 15 minutes/Cooking time – 5 minutes

For the tuna

4 fresh tuna steaks
1 tbsp olive oil for brushing
squeeze of lemon juice

For the mango salsa

1 mango (not too ripe), peeled and cut into small cubes
1 avocado (not too ripe), peeled and cut into small cubes
handful of firm cherry tomatoes, cut into quarters
1 shallot, peeled and very finely chopped
bunch of mint leaves, roughly chopped
bunch of coriander leaves, roughly chopped
½ tsp ground cumin
pinch of chilli powder

½ tsp coriander seeds, crushed in pestle and mortar
juice of 1 lime
½ tbsp extra virgin olive oil
salt and freshly ground black pepper

For the couscous
250g couscous
1 tbsp olive oil
300ml vegetable stock
75g dried cranberries

1. Prepare the mango salsa by combining all the ingredients.
2. Season and refrigerate until needed.
3. Turn on the griddle and leave it to get really hot.
4. Prepare the couscous: add a tbsp of olive oil and about 300ml stock (check pack for exact quantity of water and how long to leave it), stir and leave for 5 minutes.
5. Pour boiling water on the cranberries and leave for a few minutes to soften. Strain and stir into the couscous when it is ready, fluffing it up gently with a fork. Season the couscous according to taste.
6. When the griddle is smoking hot, brush the tuna steaks with olive oil and season with salt and black pepper and then place on the griddle for about 2 minutes each side, less if they are not very thick. They need to be pink in the middle or they will be tough.
7. Give the steaks a squeeze of lemon or lime juice, season with more salt and pepper and serve on individual plates with the couscous and the salsa.

Lebanese Couscous Salad with Griddled Vegetables and a Spiced Yoghurt Sauce

Excellent balanced, healthy, low-fat vegetarian meal, good for training.

I often make a large amount of this salad and keep it in the fridge to snack on when I am training. It keeps for two to three days in the fridge and the flavours seem to improve over this time. It is not only packed with vitamins from the herbs and vegetables, but the couscous is a good low-fat, slow-burning carbohydrate. Wholemeal couscous is really good, although not always available in the supermarket. I buy mine from the local health food shop. If you are planning to go to the gym after work, put a tub of this in your lunch box. It also makes a good vegetarian evening meal, or an accompaniment to a piece of grilled chicken or a lamb chop.

Nutrition per serving

Energy (kcal)	435	Protein (g)	14
Carbohydrate (g)	58	Fat (g)	18
Of which sugars (g)	11	Of which saturates (g)	3
Salt (g)	0.7	Fibre (g)	5

Serves 4

Prep time – 10 minutes/Cooking time – 10 minutes

For the couscous

250g couscous (wholemeal if you can get it)
4 tbsp good olive oil plus 1 tbsp to soak the couscous
plenty of salt and pepper
1 tsp ground coriander
large bunch of flat-leaf parsley, roughly chopped
large bunch of mint leaves, roughly chopped
6 spring onions, finely sliced
4 tomatoes, chopped up small
4 tbsp lemon juice
small handful of pomegranate seeds or toasted pine nuts for decoration

For the griddled vegetables

2 large courgettes, sliced lengthways with a sharp knife to about ½cm thickness
1 aubergine, sliced lengthways with a sharp knife to about ½cm thickness
½ tbsp balsamic vinegar
2 tbsp good olive oil

For the yoghurt sauce

250g natural low fat yoghurt
½ tsp ground cumin
½ tsp coriander
¼ tsp chilli powder
salt and freshly ground pepper
small clove of garlic, crushed
handful mint leaves, chopped

1. Put the couscous in a bowl with a pinch of salt and a tbsp of olive oil. Pour over 300ml boiling water and leave for about 5 minutes (check the pack for exact amount of water and time).
2. Heat a griddle or frying pan. Brush the courgettes and aubergine with the olive oil and cook on each side for a few minutes (so that nice stripes appear).
3. When the couscous is ready, fluff it up with a fork and then add the herbs, spring onions, tomatoes, ground coriander, lemon juice and the rest of the olive oil. Taste and add salt and pepper accordingly.
4. Mix the yoghurt sauce ingredients together, pour into a bowl and gently pour a little fruity olive oil around the edge of the bowl.
5. On a large platter, arrange the aubergine and courgette slices around the edge, dress with the balsamic vinegar and 1 tbsp olive oil and then pile the couscous into the middle. Decorate with pomegranate seeds or pine nuts and serve with the yoghurt sauce.

Aromatic Chickpea Couscous with Grilled Sea Bream, Salsa Verde and Roasted Tomatoes

Omega-3 fatty acids, low-G.I. carbohydrate, protein and plenty of vitamins make this meal perfect for training.

This is one of my failsafe dinner party dishes. It is elegant but really easy to cook and it provides a good balance of nutrients to keep you going on your training run the following morning. The salsa verde is just packed with vitamins and omega-3 fatty acids and is absolutely delicious with any grilled fish – you can use sea bass, mackerel or tuna just as successfully.

Nutrition per serving

Energy (kcal)	750	Protein (g)	56
Carbohydrate (g)	67	Fat (g)	31
Of which sugars (g)	9	Of which saturates (g)	4
Salt (g)	3.7	Fibre (g)	8

Serves 4

Prep time – 10 minutes/Cooking time – 10 minutes

For the sea bream and tomatoes

Small tomatoes on the vine – 4 stems

2 tbsp olive oil

1 tbsp balsamic vinegar

4 sea bream, filleted so you get two fillets each

For the salsa verde

3 tbsp flat-leaf parsley, roughly chopped

1 tbsp fresh mint, roughly chopped

6 small anchovy filets, chopped small

3 tbsp capers

1 clove of garlic, peeled and crushed

1 tbsp Dijon mustard

juice of ½ a lemon or 2 tbsp white wine vinegar

8 tbsp extra virgin olive oil
salt and freshly ground black pepper

For the couscous
250g couscous (wholemeal if you can get it)
1 tsp salt
2 tbsp olive oil
1 x 400g tin of chickpeas, rinsed and drained
½ tsp ras-el-hanout powder (or Moroccan spice mix)

1. Preheat the oven to 180°C/gas mark 4.
2. Prepare the salsa verde – combine all the ingredients except the salt together in a blender or with a pestle and mortar until you have quite a coarse mixture. You may want to add salt afterwards depending on the saltiness of the anchovies.
3. Brush a baking tray with a little olive oil and gently lay out the tomato stems. Drizzle with a little more oil and season with salt and pepper. Roast in the oven for about 10 minutes until the tomatoes start to soften. Take them out of the oven and pour over 1 tbsp of good balsamic vinegar.
4. Meanwhile prepare the couscous – rinse in cold water and then place in a bowl with the salt and the olive oil. Pour over 300ml boiling water and leave for 5 minutes (check pack for exact quantity of water and how long to leave it). Warm the chickpeas in a small saucepan with a tbsp olive oil. When the couscous is ready, fluff it up gently with a fork, adding the chickpeas and the ras-el-hanout as you do so.
5. Heat the grill to hot. Brush the fish with a little oil and season generously with salt and pepper. Lay the fillets out on a grilling tray, skin side up. Place the tray under the grill and grill the fish for about 5 minutes, until the skin becomes nice and crisp. Move the grill tray to the oven and bake for another couple of minutes, until the fish is just cooked through.
6. Serve on warmed plates – place two fillets on each plate with a generous spoonful of salsa verde, a stem of tomatoes and the couscous.

Turkish Turlu Turlu with Couscous and Tahini Sauce

Low-G.I., high-carbohydrate meal, great for endurance and general training.

This is an excellent vegetarian main course or accompaniment to grilled chicken kebabs or a piece of fish. You basically slow-roast any vegetables you might have in your vegetable rack with spices and olive oil. It is especially good with vegetables that will caramelise nicely in the oven – root vegetables like turnips, beetroot, carrots and onions, for instance, mixed with Mediterranean vegetables like peppers and aubergines. The addition of the chickpeas makes the meal more substantial and adds the all-important iron factor which is often missing in vegetarian food. Tahini is a thick paste made from sesame seeds, most commonly used with chickpeas to make hummus. Not only does it make a delicious sauce, but it is packed with vital minerals such as copper, magnesium and calcium. This dish is also good sprinkled with roughly broken pieces of feta cheese.

Nutrition per serving

Energy (kcal)	676	Protein (g)	20
Carbohydrate (g)	58	Fat (g)	40
Of which sugars (g)	16	Of which saturates (g)	7
Salt (g)	3.2	Fibre (g)	14

Serves 4

Prep time – 10–15 minutes/Cooking time – 45 minutes

For the Turlu turlu

2 courgettes

1 aubergine

1 green pepper

1 red pepper

3–4 waxy new potatoes

2 medium turnips

1 onion, peeled and cut into thick slices
1 fennel bulb, cut into thick slices
4 cloves of garlic, peeled, 2 crushed and 2 whole
6 tbsp extra virgin olive oil
1 tbsp coriander seeds, crushed with a pestle and mortar
1 tsp cumin seeds, crushed with a pestle and mortar
1 tsp ground allspice
plenty of salt and freshly ground black pepper
1 x 400g can of chickpeas, drained
250ml passata (about ½ jar)
large handful of herbs (flat-leaf parsley and coriander, or fresh thyme and oregano), roughly chopped

For the couscous
250g couscous (wholemeal if you can get it)
1 tsp salt
knob of butter

For the tahini sauce
2 cloves of garlic, peeled
large pinch of salt
3 tbsp tahini
juice of 1 lemon
6 tbsp water
salt and freshly ground black pepper
1 tbsp extra virgin olive oil

1. Preheat the oven to 200°C/gas mark 6.
2. Chop up all the vegetables into 2–3cm chunks and put them all into a bowl with the olive oil, the crushed garlic, whole garlic, the spices and some salt and pepper. Mix together so that the vegetables are coated with the oil mix.
3. Lay the vegetables (except the courgettes) onto a really big roasting tray so that they form one layer and pop them into the oven for about 40–45 minutes or until they start to caramelise. Turn the vegetables every now and then. Stir in the courgettes after about 35 minutes.

4. While the vegetables are cooking, prepare the couscous and the tahini sauce.
5. For the couscous, rinse grains in cold water and then place in a bowl with the salt and the butter. Pour over 300ml boiling water and leave for 5 minutes (check pack for exact quantity of water and how long to leave it). Fluff up gently with a fork.
6. For the tahini sauce, pound the garlic and salt to a paste with a pestle and mortar, put into a bowl with the tahini paste and whisk in the lemon juice. Gradually whisk in about 6 tbsp water, until you have a thick creamy sauce. Add salt and pepper and then drizzle with the olive oil.
7. Heat up the passata and the chickpeas in a pan, then gently stir into the vegetables. Bake for a further 5 minutes.
8. Add the herbs, check for seasoning and serve with the couscous and the tahini sauce.

lentils and pulses

'I particularly need to keep an eye on my iron levels. I don't/can't eat red meat but luckily I adore spinach and lentils, so if I really need a boost I make daal for dinner.' Melissa, gofasterfood blog contributor.

Chickpea Falafel

Delicious and healthy low-G.I. snack or light meal.

I love to eat falafel for lunch or as a light supper, perhaps followed by a bowl of soup. They have been a staple in the Middle Eastern diet for centuries and are either eaten on their own, as part of a mezze or tucked into pitta bread with salad, tomatoes and usually tahini or yoghurt sauce (see page 205).

Nutrition per serving

Energy (kcal)	305	Protein (g)	18
Carbohydrate (g)	49	Fat (g)	5.5
Of which sugars (g)	11	Of which saturates (g)	1
Salt (g)	4	Fibre (g)	7

Serves 2
Prep time – 10 minutes + 30 minutes in fridge/ Cooking time – 10 minutes

280g tinned chickpeas, drained
juice of ½ a lemon
2 cloves of garlic peeled and chopped
1 tsp ground cumin
1 tsp ground coriander
½ tsp cayenne pepper
1 fresh green chilli, deseeded and finely chopped
1 dessertspoon tahini (optional)
1 tsp salt
50g plain flour
1 tsp baking powder
2 tbsp fresh parsley, chopped
1 tbsp fresh mint, chopped
rapeseed, groundnut or sunflower oil for frying

1. Mix together the chickpeas with the lemon juice, garlic, cumin, coriander, cayenne, fresh chilli, tahini and salt and puree with a food processor or hand-held blender.
2. Add the flour, the baking powder and the chopped herbs and mix together.
3. Roll the mixture into little balls the size of a walnut (about 3cm in diameter) and let them set in the fridge for 30 minutes.
4. Heat some oil in a non-stick frying pan to fry the falafel – you need quite a lot of oil, to cover the pan by ½cm in depth. When the oil is nice and hot, place the balls into the oil, push them gently down with a spoon to form little patties. Fry them gently for about 4 minutes on each side, so that they form a golden crust. You may need to do this in batches. Remove and place on a piece of kitchen paper to eliminate any excess oil.
5. Serve the falafel with the yoghurt or the tahini sauce (see page 205), some lemon wedges and, if you like, a herby salad.

Sweet potato, Courgette and Coriander Koftas

Delicious and healthy low-G.I. snack or light meal.

Eat these as you would falafel, as a starter or light midweek meal, accompanied by yoghurt or tahini sauce (see page 205).

Nutrition per serving

Energy (kcal)	181	Protein (g)	9
Carbohydrate (g)	28	Fat (g)	4.5
Of which sugars (g)	2.5	Of which saturates (g)	0.5
Salt (g)	1.2	Fibre (g)	5

Serves 4
Prep time – 20 minutes + 30 minutes in fridge/
Cooking time – 5 minutes

1 small sweet potato, peeled and diced
1 tsp cumin seeds
1 tsp coriander seeds
1 x 400g can of chickpeas
2cm cube fresh ginger, peeled and grated
1 tbsp lemon juice
1 clove of garlic, peeled and crushed
½ tsp salt
2 tbsp flour
1 courgette, finely grated
freshly ground black pepper
good-sized handful fresh coriander and/or mint leaves, chopped
2 tbsp sunflower or rapeseed oil

1. Boil the sweet potato in plenty of salted water for about 10 minutes until just tender, then drain.
2. Dry fry the cumin and coriander seeds for 1 minute and then roughly crush them with a pestle and mortar.
3. Put the chickpeas, sweet potato, spices, lemon juice, garlic, fresh

ginger, salt and pepper into a food processor and blend until semi-puréed.

4. Mix in the flour, the courgette and the chopped coriander and/or mint.
5. Form little patties about 3cm in diameter and 1cm thick and leave in the fridge for 30 minutes to become firm.
6. Heat 2 tablespoons of sunflower or rapeseed oil in a non-stick frying pan and fry the patties for 2 minutes on each side.
7. Serve with yoghurt or tahini sauce.

Yoghurt sauce for falafel and koftas

½ tsp cumin
½ tsp ground coriander
¼ tsp chilli powder
250g low-fat natural yoghurt

Combine the ingredients together in a bowl and chill until needed.

Tahini sauce for falafel and koftas

2 cloves of garlic
large pinch of salt
juice of 1 lemon
3 tbsp tahini
6 tbsp water
salt and freshly ground black pepper
1 tbsp extra virgin olive oil

Pound the garlic and salt to a paste with a pestle and mortar, put into a bowl with the tahini and whisk in the lemon juice. Gradually whisk in the water, until you have a thick creamy sauce. Add salt and pepper and then drizzle with the olive oil.

Fabada Asturiana or Asturian Bean Stew

Comfort food at its best – great to warm you up and replace lost calories after a cold and wet cycle ride, run or swim in the sea.

Fabada is a deliciously rich bean stew, orginating from the Asturias region of northern Spain. My mother used to cook this on cold days when I was a child and it has been a favourite of mine ever since. It is one of those dishes where you can just throw all the ingredients in a pot and then pop the pot into the oven for hours. It is perfect for midweek if you have people coming in and out, kids doing various sporting activities, all eating at different times – this happens quite frequently in our household. This meal is ideal for carbo-loading or to hit the spot after a big training session. The idea is that it is chunky, so don't worry about chopping the vegetables carefully. It is best to use beans that have been soaked overnight for this dish.

Nutrition per serving

Energy (kcal)	663	Protein (g)	30
Carbohydrate (g)	35	Fat (g)	45
Of which sugars (g)	11	Of which saturates (g)	12
Salt (g)	2.5	Fibre (g)	12

Serves 4
Prep time – 10 minutes + overnight soaking for beans/
Cooking time – 3 hours

300g butter beans, soaked overnight and then drained and rinsed
1 whole chorizo sausage or two small ones (about 150g), cut into large chunks
4 pieces of pork belly (about 700g) cut into large 4cm chunks
250g bacon misshapes
3 cloves of garlic, peeled and crushed
2 bay leaves
a few sprigs of thyme
1 onion, peeled and roughly chopped
1 leek, roughly chopped

3 sticks celery, roughly chopped
2 red peppers, roughly chopped
2 carrots, peeled and roughly chopped
10 peppercorns
1 x 400g tin chopped tomatoes
100g (small tin) tomato puree
1 tsp Spanish smoked paprika
1 tsp ground cumin
1 tsp ground coriander
1 tsp ras-el-hanout
salt and freshly ground black pepper
large glug of olive oil
plenty of chopped flat-leaf parsley to serve

1. Drain the beans and place them in a large, heavy-bottomed casserole dish. Just cover them with cold water, bring to the boil and cook rapidly for about 10 minutes. Remove any scum with a slotted spoon.
2. Then add the rest of the ingredients (except the salt and parsley) and top up with enough fresh water to cover everything to a depth of 2.5cm.
3. Bring to the boil again and then turn down the heat so that it is very low, cover and simmer for 2½–3 hours, until the beans are quite soft and the meat is tender. The simmering needs to be really gentle – use a diffuser to keep the heat really low, or put the pot in the oven at 150–160°C/gas mark 2–3 instead. Have a look after a couple of hours and add more water if necessary. Try to shake the casserole rather than stir it so that the beans do not break. Skim off any excess fat from the surface.
4. About 10 minutes before the fabada is ready, add salt (do not add salt before or it makes the beans go tough) and pepper. Taste – you may want to add some extra spice.
5. Serve sprinkled with fresh parsley, and with chunks of crusty granary bread.

Flageolet and Chickpea Soup

Beans and pulses are a very healthy low-G.I. carbohydrate and chickpeas are rich in manganese, which is very good for your bones.

Although this soup conjures up autumnal images, I have to say that I last made it on a July evening in the South of France with some leftover lamb stock. We ate it on the terrace and mopped up the juices with some crusty French bread. This soup is a meal in itself, it is very easy to make and is great for endurance. You can experiment with different types of bean – flageolet and chickpeas work really well together, but you might want to try butter beans or borlotti beans in place of the chickpeas.

Nutrition per serving

Energy (kcal)	313	Protein (g)	16
Carbohydrate (g)	44	Fat (g)	9
Of which sugars (g)	17	Of which saturates (g)	1
Salt (g)	2	Fibre (g)	12

Serves 4
Prep time – 5 minutes/Cooking time – 20–25 minutes

1 tbsp olive oil
2 onions or 2 leeks, or 1 of each, sliced
2 bay leaves
2 carrots, peeled and roughly chopped
2 celery stalks, roughly chopped
2 tsp paprika
2 tsp ras-el-hanout spice mix
1 cinnamon stick
2 cloves of garlic, peeled and crushed
2cm piece of fresh ginger, peeled and grated
grated zest of two oranges
1 x 400g tin of flageolet beans
1 x 400g tin of chickpeas

2 x 400g tin of chopped tomatoes
2 tbsp tomato puree
1 litre good chicken or lamb stock
large handful of flat-leaved parsley or coriander leaves, chopped roughly
extra virgin olive oil to serve

1. In a large pan, gently sauté the onions and/or leeks in olive oil with the bay leaves for about 5 minutes until translucent.
2. Add the carrots and celery to the pan and cook for 5 minutes or so.
3. Add the spices.
4. Add the garlic, ginger, orange zest, beans and chickpeas, tomatoes, tomato puree and the stock.
5. Cover and simmer gently for about 10–15 minutes until the vegetables are tender. Check for seasoning. You may need some more spice – play around a bit; you could try adding a little ground coriander or cardamom, for instance. Add the fresh herbs, reserving some for decoration.
6. Transfer to a large serving bowl. Drizzle some fruity olive oil onto the soup and sprinkle with a little fresh parsley or coriander.
7. Eat with chunks of crusty bread.

Puy Lentils with Grilled Organic Sausages

Due to their high soluble fibre content, lentils are digested very slowly and can really help towards maintaining stable blood glucose levels – great for keeping you going until the next meal or through your workout.

This puy lentil salad is incredibly easy to make and is the perfect accompaniment to sausages. A much healthier alternative to sausages and mash for us athletes, it is also quicker and much less messy to make. Puy lentils, also known as green lentils, require no soaking and absorb the flavours they are cooked with extremely well. They have a low G.I. and they are high in fibre, protein, vitamin B1 and minerals, especially iron and magnesium. I buy my sausages from my local farm shop. They are tasty, have a high meat content and are not too salty. If you are buying supermarket sausages, get the posh organic ones, or the ones with the highest meat content you can afford ... it makes a real difference. You can find jars of preserved semi-dried, or sunblush, tomatoes on the antipasto shelf in the supermarket. They are fantastic added to pasta sauces or even just to snack on with an aperitif. They melt in the mouth and have an intense, fruity flavour, a hundred times more delicious than the more leathery sun-dried tomatoes.

Nutrition per serving

Energy (kcal)	605	Protein (g)	18
Carbohydrate (g)	28	Fat (g)	47
Of which sugars (g)	6	Of which saturates (g)	14
Salt (g)	2	Fibre (g)	4

Serves 4
Prep time – 2 minutes/Cooking time – 30 minutes

For the sausages and lentils
8 good-quality organic sausages
300g puy lentils
1 onion, peeled and studded with 5 or 6 cloves

2 cloves of garlic
3 bay leaves
1 tsp red wine vinegar
1 tsp sugar

For the dressing
2 tbsp red wine vinegar
4 tbsp extra virgin olive oil
salt and freshly ground black pepper
1 tsp ground coriander
handful of flat-leaf parsley, chopped
squeeze of lemon
10 semi-dried/sunblush tomatoes

1. Rinse the lentils in cold water and put them in a pan with the onion and cloves, garlic, bay leaves, a teaspoon of red wine vinegar and a teaspoon of sugar.
2. Pour in cold water so that it covers the lentils by 2cm.
3. Cover and bring to the boil. Boil rapidly for 10 minutes and then simmer for a further 20 minutes, until the lentils are tender. I like them to have a bit of a bite to them still.
4. Meanwhile grill your sausages.
5. When the lentils are cooked, discard the onion and the bay leaves, and stir in the dressing ingredients, with plenty of salt and pepper to taste.
6. Serve warm with the sausages.
7. A crisp green salad is a perfect accompaniment to this dish.

Slow-cooked Lamb with Flageolet Beans

Brimming with nutrition, good for both endurance and post-exercise recovery.

Flageolet beans are immature kidney beans, pale green in colour or sometimes white. They are very tender and have a lovely light, fresh taste. And of course they are healthy and great for endurance. They contain a decent amount of protein and fibre, about 65 per cent low G.I. carbohydrate and they are rich in minerals, especially calcium, potassium and magnesium. This lamb dish is a fantastic thing to cook on a Saturday, to eat the evening before your long Sunday endurance session or to recover from your Saturday workout. Serve it with couscous or pasta or with crushed new potatoes with garlic and parsley, or just plain mashed potatoes. You can leave it in the oven for hours, it makes the house smell delicious and it is good enough for a supper party. In fact, I managed to feed 20 running friends with this after the Bristol Half Marathon – I made the dish the day before until step 4, ran the half marathon on the Sunday morning, raced back and then had time to finish it off and to squeeze in a quick shower before everyone arrived. A dollop of green garlic sauce is lovely on top.

Nutrition per serving

Energy (kcal)	600	Protein (g)	46
Carbohydrate (g)	25	Fat (g)	32
Of which sugars (g)	8	Of which saturates (g)	10
Salt (g)	1.4	Fibre (g)	8

Serves 6

Prep time – 10 minutes (plus overnight soaking if using dried beans)/Cooking time – 2¼ hours

For the lamb and beans

1 kg lamb neck fillet or shoulder, cut into 2cm cubes
2 tbsp flour
salt and freshly ground black pepper
2 tbsp olive oil

2 onions or leeks, finely sliced
2 cloves garlic, crushed
2 cloves garlic, finely sliced
2 carrots, peeled and cut into 3cm sticks
1 stick celery, finely chopped
2 anchovy fillets, finely chopped
3 bay leaves
300ml lamb stock, or enough to cover the meat
300ml dry white wine
1 bouquet garni
4 fresh thyme sprigs
225g flageolet beans, soaked overnight (or 2 x 400g tins)
300g cherry tomatoes

For the green garlic sauce
½ bulb of garlic, separated into cloves and peeled
½ tsp salt
½ tsp cumin
25ml white wine vinegar
handful of fresh parsley or coriander leaves
1 egg yolk
100ml olive oil

1. Preheat the oven to 140°C/gas mark 1.
2. Use a casserole dish that you can put on the hob and in the oven. Toss the meat in a couple of tablespoons of seasoned flour. Heat up a tablespoon of oil in the casserole dish and brown the lamb over a high heat, a few pieces at a time, then set aside on a plate.
3. Add the remaining oil to the pan and then gently sauté the onion or leek for a few minutes until golden. Add the garlic, carrots, celery, anchovies and bay leaves and fry for a minute, then return the meat to the dish and add the stock and wine, the bouquet garni and the thyme. If you are using dried beans which you have soaked overnight, add them at this stage (discarding the soaking water). If you are using tinned beans, then they will need to be added later with the tomatoes or they will go mushy.

4. Give everything a good stir, bring it up to the boil, add a few grinds of black pepper and put the dish into the oven to simmer gently for 1½ hours.
5. After this time, add the cherry tomatoes (and the tinned beans if using) and cook for a further ½ hour.
6. Before serving, check for seasoning and add salt and pepper if necessary.
7. To make the garlic sauce, puree the garlic, salt, cumin and vinegar in a blender or pestle and mortar. Add the fresh parsley and blend again.
8. In a clean bowl, whisk the egg yolk with the parsley mixture and then gradually add the oil, whisking all the time until the sauce thickens. Put a dollop onto each plate when you serve the lamb.

Smoky Black Bean and Chorizo Chilli with Salsa

High-energy, low-G.I. meal, packed with nutrients.

'All I want is black bean soup and you to make it with me'. Anyone old enough to have enjoyed *Starsky and Hutch* as a child might remember this song as one of David Soul's very few, rather dubious hits. Anyway, I always sing it in my head when I think about this dish. There is something very convivial about a bowl of chilli and this is a wonderfully tasty alternative to your common or garden chilli, easy to cook up for something like bonfire night – just double the quantities to make a big vat of the stuff. It is also really, really healthy. Black beans are high in protein and are a very good source of fibre, complex low-G.I. carbohydrate, B vitamins, iron, calcium and other minerals. They are also loaded with antioxidants and studies have shown that, gram for gram, they contain 10 times more antioxidants than oranges. You can buy them dried and tinned in most supermarkets. Serve this chilli in warmed soup bowls with a dollop of salsa on top and a chunk of crusty bread, or with some brown basmati rice and green garlic sauce (see Slow-cooked lamb with flageolet beans, page 212).

Nutrition per serving

Energy (kcal)	534	Protein (g)	38
Carbohydrate (g)	36	Fat (g)	27
Of which sugars (g)	12	Of which saturates (g)	4
Salt (g)	2	Fibre (g)	8

Serves 4
Prep time – 10 minutes + overnight soaking/
Cooking time – 1½ hours

For the smoky chilli

400g stewing beef, chopped into fairly small chunks (1cm)
2 tbsp flour mixed with ¼ tsp each salt, pepper and cayenne pepper
2 tbsp olive oil
100g chorizo chopped into 1cm chunks

1 onion, peeled and sliced finely
2 green peppers, deseeded and chopped into 1cm chunks
1 bay leaf
1 tsp smoked paprika
1 large clove of garlic, peeled and crushed
100g black beans, rinsed and soaked overnight, then rinsed again and drained (you can use tinned as an alternative, but the dried beans will be superior in both taste and texture)
500ml chicken stock
1 x 400g tin of chopped tomatoes
handful of chopped coriander leaves
squeeze of lime juice
1 green chilli, finely sliced and with seeds remaining, or two if you like it really hot

For the salsa
½ small cucumber
1 avocado, peeled
10 cherry tomatoes
4 spring onions
1 tsp coriander seed, crushed in pestle and mortar
handful of mint leaves, roughly chopped
handful of coriander leaves, roughly chopped
juice of 1 lime
glug of olive oil

1. Preheat the oven to 160°C/gas mark 3.
2. Use a casserole dish that you can put on the hob and in the oven. Toss the meat in the flour mix. Heat up a tablespoon of oil in the casserole dish and brown the beef in batches over a high heat. Set the beef aside and then quickly brown the chorizo and set aside. Scrape the juices off the bottom of the pan. A good way to do this is to pour a splash of whisky or brandy in and the brown scrapings come off the bottom of the pan really easily. Pour the juices onto the beef.
3. Add the remaining oil and then gently sauté the onion and green

pepper with the bay leaf for a few minutes. Add the smoked paprika and stir. Add the garlic, the meat, the black beans, the stock and the tin of tomatoes and bring it all to the boil.

4. Give everything a good stir and then transfer to the oven and simmer for 1½ hours until the beef and the beans are tender and the sauce has become nice and thick.
5. Add the coriander and lime juice and taste for seasoning. You might want to add some salt and pepper at this stage or a little more smoked paprika.
6. Make the salsa by chopping up the avocado, cucumber and tomatoes very small and mixing them with the other ingredients. Don't make it too far in advance as it is best really fresh.
7. Serve the chopped green chillies in a bowl on the side for people to sprinkle over the top of the chilli to their own taste.

Warm Salad of Seared Tuna with White Beans

A healthy balanced meal, ideal for summer training, high in omega-3 fatty acids, vitamins, protein, minerals and low-G.I. carbohydrate. White beans are good for endurance and are a nice alternative low-G.I. carbohydrate to rice and pasta.

Fresh tuna is truly delicious and is particularly high in omega-3 fatty acids, vitamins, protein and minerals. In fact, it is so good for you, it would be impossible to list all the reasons why in a small space. It is very important to buy it really fresh and use it on the day you buy it. Also don't overcook it as it will turn into a tasteless rubber lump! Wait until the pan is extremely hot and just sear it on both sides for a minute or so. If you can't get hold of fresh tuna, a piece of salmon fillet is a good alternative. The white beans are a good source of fibre, protein, potassium, iron and other minerals. We really should eat them more often.

Nutrition per serving

Energy (kcal)	509	Protein (g)	35
Carbohydrate (g)	20	Fat (g)	33
Of which sugars (g)	2	Of which saturates (g)	7
Salt (g)	2.5	Fibre (g)	4

Serves 4
Prep time – 5 minutes/Cooking time – 10 minutes

100g pancetta cubes
2 tbsp olive oil
2 cloves of garlic, peeled and crushed
2 x 400g cans of butter beans
4 semi-dried/sunblush tomatoes, chopped (use fresh tomatoes as an alternative)
2 tbsp lemon juice
large handful flat-leaf parsley, chopped
2 tbsp balsamic vinegar

4 tbsp extra virgin olive oil
2 preserved lemons, sliced very finely, pulp removed, plus a little of the brine for the dressing
bunch of rocket and/or spinach
salt and freshly ground black pepper to taste
4 thick tuna steaks

1. Sauté the pancetta gently in a tbsp of the olive oil for five minutes until cooked. Add the garlic, white beans, tomatoes, lemon juice and half of the parsley and heat through. Season with salt and pepper.
2. Make the dressing by mixing together the balsamic vinegar, 4 tbsp of extra virgin olive oil, the preserved lemon, the rest of the parsley, salt, pepper and the preserved lemon brine (1–2 tsp) to taste. Arrange the rocket and/or spinach on 4 plates (it looks good in really large flat-bottomed pasta bowls) and spoon on a little of the white bean mixture.
3. Lightly brush the tuna with a little olive oil and heat the griddle pan or frying pan. When it is really hot, fry the steaks for a couple of minutes on each side. Don't overcook them. They should be pink inside and they will continue to cook slightly after you have removed them from the pan.
4. Place a steak on top of each bed of white beans and generously drizzle over the dressing.

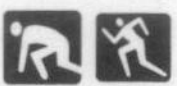

Welsh Cawl with Pearl Barley

Warming and sustaining for general training.

We spent one Spring Bank Holiday weekend camping on a totally idyllic farm on the Pembrokeshire coast. I was training for the 15 mile Brecon Beacons 3 Peaks fell run at the time and had wonderful and ambitious plans of running up and down the coast path. Unfortunately the weather was so wild, windy and rainy that the thought of coming back for a cold wash at the sink in the middle of the field (no hot showers available at this campsite, unfortunately) was enough to deter me. We spent a lot of time sheltering in the local pub instead which fortunately served a good local brew and the most wonderful Welsh cawl, a hearty stew of tender lamb and root vegetables. This is my version – the addition of pearl barley may not be particularly authentic, but it certainly adds fibre, vitamins and minerals to an already healthy, low-G.I. meal. This is quite a plain dish, so it is important to be generous with the seasoning and fresh herbs.

Nutrition per serving

Energy (kcal)	422	Protein (g)	36
Carbohydrate (g)	37	Fat (g)	15
Of which sugars (g)	9	Of which saturates (g)	7
Salt (g)	0.8	Fibre (g)	6

Serves 6

Prep time – 5 mins/Cooking time – 2 hours

900g stewing lamb – best end of neck cutlets, excess fat removed, cut into large chunks
2 tbsp oil
12 peppercorns
2 bay leaves
2 sprigs of thyme
1 large parsnip, peeled, whole
100g pearl barley
1 onion, peeled, whole

4 waxy potatoes, peeled and chopped into bite-size chunks
1 small swede, peeled and chopped into bite-size chunks
3 carrots, peeled and chopped into bite-size chunks
3 leeks, peeled and chopped into bite-size chunks
1 lamb stock cube
bunch of fresh flat-leaf parsley, or pack of mixed fresh herbs (e.g. fresh thyme, oregano, marjoram, parsley)
salt and freshly ground black pepper

1. Brown the meat in batches in a couple of tbsp of oil in a large heavy-based casserole dish.
2. Add 1½ litres of water, the onion, peppercorns, bay, thyme, the parsnip and the pearl barley.
3. Bring to the boil and then simmer, uncovered, for about 1¼ hours.
4. Remove the scum from the surface every now and then. Leave to cool so that you can spoon off the fat, which will form on the surface.
5. Remove the whole onion and the parsnip (see step 6) and any gristly bits of meat.
6. Mash the parsnip with a fork to thicken the sauce later.
7. Add the potatoes, swede and carrots to the stew and cook, covered, for a further 35 minutes.
8. Add the leeks, the mashed parsnip and the stock cube and plenty of pepper and cook for another 10 minutes.
9. Add the parsley or mixed herbs, taste for seasoning and serve in warmed bowls with crusty bread.

desserts, cakes and energy bars

'We had a pannier stuffed with energy bars which we would gobble down throughout the day!' Mavis Paterson a.k.a. Grannymave, 70, retired nurse, long-distance cyclist and runner. Best event – 4,500 mile transcontinental bike ride across Canada, 2008.

'My goodness me, your puddings are delicious! Just as tasty as a large steamed treacle pudding and lashings of custard – but 10 times more nutritious I reckon, and so much less of a burden on the long 10 milers!' Mark Collingwood, solicitor, marathon runner (personal best: 3:24). Best event – Amsterdam Marathon 2006.

'A big no-no for me is any kind of gel. I'm definitely in favour of keeping it simple, maybe some banana or fruit bar.' Carolyn Forsyth, housewife, mother, marathon runner (personal best: 3:13). Best event – Davos Alpine Marathon.

'What do I remember about my marathon training diet? I ate an awful lot of flapjacks.' Bruce Hodgson, company owner, completed New York and Amsterdam marathons (personal best: 4:12, Amsterdam 2006).

'Post race means big carbo- and sugar-loading for me – Starbucks coffee and cakes' Sally O'Grady, mother, company director. Best events: Mendip Muddle (20km multi-terrain) and Dublin Marathon (personal best: 3:52, 2008).

Almond Tarta di Santiago

Good energy food, a great treat for after exercise or for a nutritious dessert, as well as gluten-free.

This fantastic almond cake comes from Santiago de Compostela, the capital of one of my favourite areas of Spain, Galicia. It is named after the patron saint of Spain, St James, and is traditionally made with just almonds, sugar and eggs. Sometimes it has a sweet pastry case, but my version is without pastry. It is not only more virtuous as it contains absolutely no butter, but it is moist and light, gluten-free and a great natural energy food. The almonds in this cake provide good, cholesterol-reducing monounsaturated fats and also contain significant amounts of the antioxidant vitamin E, plus magnesium and potassium. It is also an incredibly quick cake to make and good enough to serve up as a dessert with a dollop of cream or some fruit.

Nutrition per serving

Energy (kcal)	323	Protein (g)	9
Carbohydrate (g)	31	Fat (g)	18
Of which sugars (g)	30	Of which saturates (g)	2
Salt (g)	0.1	Fibre (g)	2

Makes a 23cm cake – enough for 6–8 people
Prep time – 10 minutes/Cooking time – 30–35 minutes
You will need a 23cm spring-form cake tin or flan dish, greased

4 eggs, separated
zest of 1 lemon
225g caster sugar
225g ground almonds
½ tsp cinnamon
1 tbsp medium or sweet sherry
icing sugar to decorate

1. Preheat the oven to 180°C/gas mark 4.
2. Whisk the egg whites to soft peak stage with an electric whisk.
3. Put the egg yolks, lemon zest and sugar into a separate bowl and whisk until pale and creamy.
4. Stir in the almonds, the cinnamon and the sherry.
5. Fold in the egg whites, a little at a time, and then pour the mixture into the cake tin.
6. Cook in the oven for about 30–35 minutes, until golden. If you poke a skewer into the middle of the cake, it should come out clean. Cool in the tin, on a wire rack.
7. Decorate with icing sugar.

Chocolate Panforte

Pure energy! Nutritious, keeps for months and good to nibble on before or after exercise.

Panforte is a fantastic energy food for exercise. You can squirrel it away in your cake tin and cut off a piece at a time when the mood takes you – before or after exercise or just when you fancy something sweet. It is nutritious and wholesome and you only need a tiny piece to give you a boost. Panforte is the traditional Christmas cake of Sienna. It is deliciously chewy and sticky and is packed with a combination of energy-giving nuts, dried fruit and spices. You can be quite flexible with your choice of nuts, spices and dried fruit. Just use any combination you fancy, or whatever you have in the store cupboard. The only stressful part is that you have to work very quickly once the sugar syrup is ready or the mixture stiffens and it is difficult to spread into your cake tin.

Nutrition per serving

Energy (kcal)	229	Protein (g)	4
Carbohydrate (g)	32	Fat (g)	11
Of which sugars (g)	28	Of which saturates (g)	2.5
Salt (g)	0.1	Fibre (g)	1.5

Makes a 20cm diameter cake – about 16 slices
Prep time – 15 minutes/Cooking time – 30 minutes

You will need a 20cm loose-bottomed or spring-form cake tin, greased and lined with the rice paper

3 sheets edible rice paper
80g dried fruit – I like figs and raisins, but use what you fancy
220g whole nuts – hazelnuts, Brazil and/or blanched almonds, lightly toasted
75g glacé cherries
50g crystallised ginger, chopped
75g good-quality candied peel, chopped
zest of 1 lemon

70g plain flour
2 tbsp cocoa powder
1 tsp ground cinnamon
¼ tsp ground nutmeg
¼ tsp ground coriander
¼ tsp ground cardamom
pinch of ground cloves
100g slab of dark chocolate (70 per cent cocoa)
100g sugar
115g runny honey
1 tsp orange flower water
icing sugar to dust

1. Preheat the oven to 160°C/gas mark 3.
2. Put the dried fruit, nuts, cherries, ginger, candied peel, lemon zest, flour, cocoa powder and spices into a large bowl and mix together.
3. Melt the chocolate in a separate bowl over a pan of simmering water, or in the microwave.
4. Put the sugar, honey and orange flower water into a saucepan and on a very gentle heat dissolve the sugar. When the sugar has completely dissolved, bring the mixture to the boil and boil steadily for 2 minutes.
5. Take the syrup off the heat. Combine the syrup immediately with the chocolate and then with the fruit and nut mixture. It will go all stiff but don't worry.
6. Spread it evenly into the tin, pushing it down with your fingers, and bake in the oven for 30 minutes.
7. Cool on a wire rack. Dust with icing sugar when it is cool. Cut with a very sharp knife.

FLAPJACKS AND ENERGY BARS

Flapjacks and energy bars are really good energy food, especially good for a snack on your way to a race or for straight after a big exercise session. It is important to use unrefined whole rolled oats for flapjacks and not to make them too sweet as this tends to make them less palatable and you'll find it difficult to stomach more than one. I made a variety of these bars for the journey to the London Marathon. It was a very pleasant and efficient way to carbo-load.

Date, Apricot and Walnut Flapjacks

Pre-workout, post-workout, tea-time snack ... there's always a valid excuse to eat one of these delicious and nutritious flapjacks.

Nutrition per serving

Energy (kcal)	180	Protein (g)	3
Carbohydrate (g)	18	Fat (g)	11
Of which sugars (g)	10	Of which saturates (g)	4
Salt (g)	0.1	Fibre (g)	1.5

Makes 12 flapjacks
Prep time – 5–10 minutes/Cooking time – 15–20 minutes
You will need a shallow 20cm square cake tin, lightly greased

75g butter
2 tbsp golden syrup (dip the spoon in hot water before using so the syrup is easier to pour)
1 tbsp soft light brown sugar
75g walnut pieces
75g mix of dried apricots and dates, chopped
200g whole rolled oats (unrefined porridge oats)
zest of ½ a lemon

1. Preheat the oven to 170°C/gas mark 3.
2. In a saucepan, melt the butter with the sugar and syrup on a low heat and, when the sugar has dissolved, add the fruit and nuts, lemon zest and then the porridge oats. Mix together really well. If the mixture seems sloppy, add another handful of oats.
3. Turn the mixture into the tin and press down with the back of a spoon or your fingers.
4. Bake in the oven for 15–20 minutes until golden. Remove the tin from the oven and set on a wire rack.
5. Leave to cool slightly and then mark into fingers or squares with a really sharp knife.
6. Remove the flapjacks from the tin when they are cool and firm. No doubt several will have disappeared by this time ...

Honey, Ginger and Lime Oaties

Slightly cakier than a traditional flapjack, these oaties go down a treat with everyone.

Nutrition per serving

Energy (kcal)	143	Protein (g)	2
Carbohydrate (g)	24	Fat (g)	5
Of which sugars (g)	9	Of which saturates (g)	2.5
Salt (g)	0.1	Fibre (g)	1.5

Makes 12 bars

Prep time – 5–10 minutes/Cooking time – 25 minutes

You will need a shallow 20 x 23cm cake tin, lightly greased

50g unsalted butter
1 tbsp ginger syrup (from the jar of stem ginger)
25g soft light brown sugar
2 tbsp honey
1 tbsp golden syrup
60g raisins
40g (2 lumps) stem ginger, finely chopped
zest of 1 lime, plus a good squeeze of the juice
50g self-raising flour
200g unrefined whole porridge oats

1. Pre-heat the oven to 170°C/gas mark 3.
2. Melt the butter with the sugar, honey, golden and ginger syrups on a low heat and, when the sugar has dissolved, add the raisins, ginger, lime zest and juice, the flour and then the porridge oats. Mix together really well. If the mixture seems sloppy, add another handful of oats. Turn the mixture into the tin and press down with the back of a spoon or your fingers.
3. Bake in the oven for 25 minutes until golden. Remove the tin from the oven and set on a wire rack.
4. Leave to cool slightly and then mark into fingers or squares with a very sharp knife.
5. Remove the flapjacks from the tin when they are cool and firm.

Mincemeat and Orange Flapjacks

An unusual combination of orange zest and mincemeat that really works, and doesn't need to be limited to the Christmas season.

Nutrition per serving

Energy (kcal)	375	Protein (g)	4
Carbohydrate (g)	56	Fat (g)	16
Of which sugars (g)	33	Of which saturates (g)	9
Salt (g)	0.5	Fibre (g)	3

Makes 12 bars

Prep time – 5–10 mins/Cooking time – 15–20 mins

You will need a shallow 23cm x 33cm swiss roll tin, lightly greased

175g butter
280g golden syrup
225g mincemeat
grated zest of 2 oranges
large handful of raisins
425g unrefined porridge oats

1. Pre-heat the oven to 170°C/gas mark 3.
2. Melt the butter with the syrup on a low heat. Add the mincemeat, the orange zest, the raisins and then the porridge oats. Mix together really well. If the mixture seems sloppy, add another handful of oats.
3. Turn the mixture into the tin and press down with the back of a spoon or your fingers.
4. Bake in the oven for 15–20 minutes until golden. Remove the tin from the oven and set on a wire rack.
5. Leave to cool slightly and then mark into fingers or squares with a really sharp knife.
6. Remove the flapjacks from the tin when they are cool and firm.

Malty Fruit Bars

Fantastic for both fuelling and refuelling.

These are great energy bars: soft, chewy and full of goodness. They make a superb body fuel for both before and after sport, but are equally good as a healthy afternoon snack. I got the idea of making these bars when I went to watch my husband cycle the British stage of the 2007 Tour de France – from Greenwich in London to Canterbury. Soreen Malt Loaf Bars were handed out at the snack stations during the race and they seemed to do the trick. My version includes malt extract, a fantastic high-carb sugar, which really adds to the flavour and the texture. You can get it in health food shops and big supermarkets. If you cannot find it, you could use molasses instead.

Nutrition per serving

Energy (kcal)	328	Protein (g)	5
Carbohydrate (g)	51	Fat (g)	13
Of which sugars (g)	43	Of which saturates (g)	2.5
Salt (g)	0.3	Fibre (g)	1.5

Makes 12–16 bars

Prep time – 10–15 minutes/Cooking time – 50–60 minutes

You will need a 34cm x 24cm baking tray or shallow cake tin, greased and lined

200g self-raising wholemeal flour
1 tsp ground cinnamon
1 tsp mixed spice
4 eggs
175g margarine
150g soft dark brown sugar
2 heaped tbsp malt extract
4 eggs
250g currants
175g raisins
200g sultanas

50g chopped dates
50g glacé cherries, halved
juice of 1 orange
50g walnut pieces

1. Preheat the oven to 160°C/gas mark 3.
2. Put the flour into a bowl with the spices.
3. In another bowl, cream together the margarine, the sugar and the malt extract with an electric whisk, until pale and fluffy.
4. Beat in the eggs with the whisk, one at a time, adding a spoon of flour with each of the last 3 eggs.
5. Fold in the remaining flour and then fold in the fruit and orange juice.
6. Pour the mixture into the tin and smooth the surface. Sprinkle with the nuts.
7. Bake for 50–60 minutes, until a skewer pierced through the centre comes out clean.
8. Cool on a wire rack and then cut into bars.

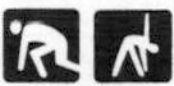

Walnut and White Chocolate Chip Brownies

High glucose content to replenish tired muscles after exercise.

It is not usually very hard to find an excuse to eat these brownies, but running is always the one I use. What is the point of running if you can't eat chocolate every now and then? It is also full of iron. These brownies just melt in your mouth and they are great for recovery. If you are not a fan of white chocolate, then use chunks of milk chocolate instead. I also sometimes use pecans or Brazil nuts instead of walnuts. These brownies make a deliciously simple dessert for a dinner party or buffet; serve with a bowl of raspberries or strawberries and a dollop of ice cream, clotted cream or crème fraîche.

Nutrition per serving

Energy (kcal)	278	Protein (g)	4
Carbohydrate (g)	28	Fat (g)	17
Of which sugars (g)	24	Of which saturates (g)	9
Salt (g)	0.4	Fibre (g)	0.5

Makes 12 brownies

Prep time – 10–15 minutes/Cooking time – 15–20 minutes

You will need a 20-23cm square cake tin, greased and lined with greaseproof paper

120g good quality dark chocolate (70 per cent cocoa)
115g softened butter
2 large eggs
150g caster sugar
1 tsp vanilla essence
20g self-raising flour
45g plain flour
1 tbsp cocoa
pinch of salt
100g white chocolate, broken into chunky pieces
50g walnuts, broken into pieces

1. Preheat the oven to 180°C/gas mark 4.
2. Put the dark chocolate into a heatproof bowl and place it over a saucepan of simmering water. When it has melted, take it off the heat, add the butter and stir it until smooth. Leave it to cool for a few minutes.
3. Break the eggs into a bowl with the sugar and vanilla essence and beat until pale and thick. Add to the melted chocolate mixture.
4. Sift the flour, salt and the cocoa into the mixture and beat it until smooth.
5. Add the white chocolate pieces and the walnuts, stir to combine and then pour the whole lot into the cake tin.
6. Bake in the oven for about 15–20 minutes. Don't overcook – the top needs to be firm but the centre needs to be gooey.
7. Leave to cool in the tin for 15 minutes or so and then cut into squares.

Chocolate Biscuit Cake

Good nutritious recovery food which will work quickly on tired muscles.

This recipe is not rocket science. In fact, any combination of dried fruit and nuts will do, but using good-quality chocolate really helps. I tend to make this cake a lot in the summer for our numerous camping trips, but it is also great recovery food for after a long exercise session. Although much loved by those with a sweet tooth, it is also a more nutritious, iron-rich and wholesome alternative to a packet of chocolate biscuits or a chocolate bar.

Nutrition per serving

Energy (kcal)	369	Protein (g)	4
Carbohydrate (g)	39	Fat (g)	22
Of which sugars (g)	29	Of which saturates (g)	11
Salt (g)	0.5	Fibre (g)	1

Makes a 20cm diameter cake – 8 slices
Prep time – 10 minutes, plus 1 hour chilling

You will need a round 20cm loose-bottomed or spring-form cake tin, lightly greased

125g plain chocolate (70 per cent cocoa), or you can use a combination of plain and good quality milk chocolate – Cadbury's Dairy Milk, for instance – for a less rich version
70g unsalted butter
1 tbsp golden syrup
1 tbsp stem ginger syrup
75g digestive biscuits, broken into small pieces
100g mix of raisins, halved glacé cherries and chopped stem ginger
50g toasted flaked almonds

1. Melt the chocolate in a bowl over a pan of simmering water, then add the butter, the golden syrup and the ginger syrup.
2. When the butter has melted, take off the heat and leave to cool slightly.
3. Add the rest of the ingredients and stir to combine.
4. Spoon out into the cake tin and flatten down.
5. Put in the fridge to chill for at least an hour.

Chocolate Pecan Tart with Cinnamon Cream

A great post-run sweet treat, super for recovery with high-G.I. golden syrup to get straight to work on your tired muscles, dark chocolate for a good iron boost, eggs for protein and delicious pecan nuts to help replace lost minerals.

Isn't it great when you can find good qualities in such a decadent treat like a sticky tart? The cinnamon cream is optional but it does give the dish that extra polish and a small dollop isn't going to do you much harm. I made this tart in advance and served it as a pudding with some strawberries for some running friends after the Forest of Dean Half Marathon. I have to say it hit the spot with everyone. The strawberries add vitamins and balance the sweetness of the tart.

Nutrition per serving

Energy (kcal)	800	Protein (g)	9
Carbohydrate (g)	103	Fat (g)	42
Of which sugars (g)	78	Of which saturates (g)	20
Salt (g)	0.8	Fibre (g)	1.5

Makes about 8 slices
Prep time for pastry – 10 minutes, plus chilling/
Cooking time – 10–12 minutes
Prep time for tart – 10 minutes/Cooking time – 40 minutes
You will need a 25cm loose-bottomed tart dish, greaseproof paper and baking beans

For the sweet pastry

1 egg
125g caster sugar
250g plain flour, sieved
125g unsalted butter, softened

For the filling
55g unsalted butter
100g dark chocolate (at least 70 per cent cocoa)
300ml golden syrup
180g granulated sugar
4 large eggs
100g pack of pecan nut halves

For the cinnamon cream
150ml whipping cream
½ tsp ground cinnamon

1. Preheat the oven to 180°C/gas mark 4.
2. To prepare the pastry, mix the egg and the sugar together in a bowl, then slowly incorporate the flour. Mix in the butter with your fingertips. Or pop it all into a food processor and let it do the work for you. Make the pastry into a ball, wrap in clingfilm and put it in the fridge for an hour.
3. Cut the pastry into thin slices and arrange on and up the sides of your tart dish, pushing each piece together gently so that it forms a flat surface – this gives you a nice thin pastry case and it is easier than rolling it out with a rolling pin. Prick the base lightly with a fork and, if you can, put it in the fridge for 30 minutes or so to settle.
4. Cover the case with greaseproof paper and line with baking beans. Bake blind in the oven for 8 minutes. Take off the greaseproof paper and bake for another 3–4 minutes.
5. Remove from the oven and cool.
6. Melt the butter and chocolate slowly in a bowl over a pan of simmering water. Stir and leave to cool a little.
7. Mix together the syrup and the sugar in a saucepan and slowly let the sugar dissolve over a low heat. When the sugar has dissolved, bring the mixture to the boil and simmer for a couple of minutes, stirring all the time. Let this cool for about 5 minutes.
8. Beat the eggs briefly with a fork and then add them to the warm chocolate mixture. Then whisk in the sugar/syrup mixture.

9. Pour the filling into the tart case and put it in the oven for about 15 minutes. When the surface of the tart is just set, arrange the pecans beautifully on top so that the whole tart is covered (I start from the outside and work into the middle).
10. Put the tart back into the oven for about 25 minutes. Put a piece of greaseproof paper over the tart to stop the pecans burning after about 10 minutes. The filling is cooked when it has risen slightly and the centre will feel set, but soft to the touch. Leave the tart to cool.
11. Whip the cream and then fold in the cinnamon and serve.

Date Tart with Cardamom and Orange Flower Water

Very high-G.I. dessert. Fantastic for refuelling after an intensive exercise session, but equally good as a stylish dessert for a dinner party.

This tart is sweet, decadent, exotic and an absolute treat. With glucose to reach your tired muscles quickly, it is great for recovery. The dates are also rich in carbohydrate, iron, potassium and other minerals which need to be replenished after a big sweaty run. There are a few unusual ingredients in this tart which make it all the more exotic – coconut cream, cardamom powder and orange flower water. You will find coconut cream in the supermarket alongside the oriental foods (Thai curry mixes, noodles, prawn crackers etc.) and orange flower water is generally found in the baking section. If you cannot find any cardamom powder, use the seeds of a cardamom pod, crushed in a pestle and mortar.

Nutrition per serving

Energy (kcal)	692	Protein (g)	6
Carbohydrate (g)	77	Fat (g)	41
Of which sugars (g)	53	Of which saturates (g)	30
Salt (g)	0.7	Fibre (g)	2

Serves about 8
Prep time for pastry – 10 minutes + chilling/
Cooking time – 10–12 minutes
Prep time for tart – 5 minutes/Cooking time – 5 minutes
You will need a 25cm loose-bottomed tart dish, greaseproof paper and baking beans

For the pastry

1 egg
125g caster sugar
250g plain flour, sieved
125g unsalted butter, softened

For the filling
100g unsalted butter
200ml golden syrup
200ml coconut cream
30 dates, sliced lengthways
1 dessertspoon dark rum
1 dessertspoon orange flower water
½ tsp cardamom powder

For the glaze
1 tbsp golden syrup
1 tbsp coconut cream

1. Turn the oven on to 180°C/gas mark 4.
2. Prepare the pastry – mix the egg and the sugar together in a bowl and the slowly incorporate the flour. Mix in the butter with your fingertips. Or pop it all into a food processor and let it do the work for you. Make the pastry into a ball, wrap in clingfilm and put it in the fridge for an hour.
3. Cut the pastry into thin slices and arrange on and up the sides of your tart dish, pushing each piece together gently so that it forms a flat surface – this gives you a nice thin pastry case and it is easier than rolling it out with a rolling pin. Prick lightly all over the base of the pastry with a fork. If you can, put it in the fridge for 30 minutes or so to settle.
4. Cover the case with greaseproof paper and line with baking beans. Bake blind in the oven for 10 minutes.
5. Prepare the filling – melt the butter with the syrup and the coconut cream in a saucepan. Stir it until the mixture bubbles.
6. Add the dates and mix them round in the syrup to make sure they are well coated. Remove the dates with a slotted spoon and arrange them on the pastry base.
7. Mix the cardamom powder, rum and orange flower water with the syrup.

8. Pour the syrup onto the dates – you just need a thin layer of syrup as you want to be able to see the glossy dates.
9. Cook in the oven for 5 minutes, until bubbling all over.
10. When the tart is slightly cooled, melt a tablespoon of golden syrup and coconut cream together until bubbling and brush the tart with this to glaze it.
11. Leave to set at room temperature; do not put it in the fridge or it will lose its gloss.
12. You could serve this with a dollop of whipped cream or crème fraîche, flavoured with a pinch of ground cardamom.

Elderflower-Poached Nectarines with Vanilla Ricotta Cream

Simple, fragrant, fresh-tasting dessert, brimming with vitamins and fibre.

Fruit is often poached in wine but this version, poached in elderflower pressé, is delicious, simple and non-alcoholic. If you are making this for a dinner party, you could try accompanying it with a glass of chilled, sweet muscat wine, but this dessert is so easy and quick you can make it for a midweek treat. You can prepare it in advance and it is good either warm or cold. You could try this recipe with peaches, pears, plums or apricots; just make sure that the fruit you use is hard, as ripe fruit will disintegrate when it is poached.

Nutrition per serving

Energy (kcal)	276	Protein (g)	7.5
Carbohydrate (g)	41	Fat (g)	10
Of which sugars (g)	35	Of which saturates (g)	6
Salt (g)	0.04	Fibre (g)	2.5

Serves 4
Prep time – 5 minutes/Cooking time – 15 minutes

For the nectarines

knob of butter
2 heaped tbsp soft dark brown sugar
6 large nectarines, halved, stone removed
300ml elderflower pressé
vanilla pod
1 tbsp cornflour

For the ricotta cream

250g ricotta
½ tsp vanilla essence

1. Beat together the ricotta and the vanilla essence in a bowl until soft and chill until needed.
2. Melt the butter and the sugar in a non-stick pan and then place the nectarines cut side down on the sugar to caramelise slightly.
3. Remove the fruit after about 3–4 minutes.
4. Add the elderflower pressé to the pan along with 300ml water and the vanilla pod and bring to the boil. Simmer the liquid for a few minutes to reduce slightly.
5. Add the fruit, cut side up, and simmer, covered, for about ten minutes until the fruit is tender.
6. Take off the heat and remove the vanilla pod. Pop the cornflour into a small dish and pour in a spoonful of the liquid. Stir until smooth and then pour the whole lot back into the pan and stir in.
7. Turn on the heat again and gently stir until the liquid thickens a little.
8. Serve either hot or cold in individual glass bowls with a dollop of the vanilla ricotta cream.

Go Faster Carrot Cake

Really moist, not too sweet, filling and packed with goodness – my all-time favourite training snack.

This cake is extremely nutritious and keeps very well. Keep it in the cake tin and snack on it whenever you are hungry. Take it to work with you and have a slice an hour before your lunchtime run.

Nutrition per serving

Energy (kcal)	588	Protein (g)	8
Carbohydrate (g)	65	Fat (g)	33
Of which sugars (g)	53	Of which saturates (g)	18
Salt (g)	1.3	Fibre (g)	3

Makes a 20cm square tin, or 23cm round tin – serves 12
Prep time – 15–20 minutes/Cooking time – 1¼ hours
You will need a 20cm square tin or 23cm round tin (springform), greased or lined with greaseproof paper

For the cake
250g unsalted butter
375g sugar (half caster, half demerara)
zest of 2 oranges
4 eggs
450g carrots, peeled and grated
100g walnuts, roughly chopped
juice of 1 orange
250g self-raising wholemeal flour, sifted
150g mix of raisins and dried cranberries
1 tsp bicarbonate of soda
1½ tsp mixed spice
1 tsp salt
small handful whole or chopped walnuts to decorate

For the icing
225g full-fat soft cheese

40g unsalted butter, at room temperature
80–100g icing sugar (depending on how sweet you like it)
squeeze of lemon or lime juice

1. Preheat the oven to 170°C/gas mark 3–4.
2. Cream the butter, sugar and orange zest together until light and fluffy.
3. Add the eggs, beating well as you add each one.
4. Fold in the grated carrots, raisins, cranberries and nuts, and add the orange juice.
5. Fold in the flour, bicarbonate of soda, spice and salt.
6. Pour into the cake tin and bake for about 1¼ hours. Baking time depends on the juiciness of the carrots, but you will know the cake is done as the cake comes away from the side of the cake tin and a skewer inserted into the middle of the cake comes out clean.
7. Turn the cake out onto a wire rack to cool.
8. Cream the cheese and butter together. Add the icing sugar and lemon juice and beat until smooth. Spread the icing generously over the cake.
9. Decorate with whole or chopped walnuts.

Orange Marmalade Cake

Lower G.I. cake, good for a pre-exercise snack.

If you like marmalade, you will love this cake. Made with bran and wholemeal flour, sultanas and nuts, it is one of those cakes that will sustain you for hours and has lovely lumps of caramelised orange from the marmalade.

Nutrition per serving

Energy (kcal)	528	Protein (g)	6
Carbohydrate (g)	52	Fat (g)	33
Of which sugars (g)	39	Of which saturates (g)	18
Salt (g)	0.7	Fibre (g)	2

Makes a 20cm round cake – serves 12

Prep time – 15 minutes/Cooking time – 1–1¼ hours

You will need a round 20cm cake tin, greased and lined well with greaseproof paper

175g unsalted butter, softened
175g demerara sugar
175g wholemeal self-raising flour
100g Sultana Bran, or Bran Flakes with a handful of sultanas
3 eggs
grated zest of 1 lemon
grated zest and juice of 1 orange
75g sultanas
2 tbsp golden syrup
3 tablespoons coarse cut marmalade
75g chopped walnuts or pecans (for a healthier option), with a few saved for decoration

For the icing

400g cream cheese
100g icing sugar
zest of ½ orange or lemon (plus some for decoration)

1. Preheat the oven to 180°C/gas mark 4.
2. Cream the butter and sugar until light and fluffy.
3. Crush the Sultana Bran or Bran Flakes.
4. Beat in the eggs, and then fold in the flour, lemon and orange zest, orange juice, crushed Sultana Bran, sultanas, chopped nuts, marmalade and golden syrup. You need the consistency to be quite loose so add some more juice if it is a bit too solid.
5. Spoon into the tin and level out the surface. Place in the oven for about 1–1¼ hours. The cake should be springy to the touch. Cool on a wire rack.
6. Combine the cheese, icing sugar and orange or lemon zest until smooth and then spread evenly over the top of the cake. Decorate with grated orange zest and/or some walnuts.

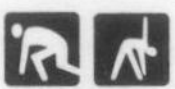

Mint and Pineapple Carpaccio

Good for recovery – rehydrating, refreshing and high in natural sugar.

This is a very simple, fruity version of the traditional beef carpaccio, which you could serve as a dessert or a starter or even as an accompaniment to a piece of fish or a pork chop. I think it is a lovely pudding to serve after an oriental dish like a Thai curry with fragrant jasmine rice. Pineapple has many qualities which are beneficial to the runner – it is high in vitamin C and it is thought to have anti-inflammatory and healing qualities.

Nutrition per serving

Energy (kcal)	92	Protein (g)	1.5
Carbohydrate (g)	18	Fat (g)	2
Of which sugars (g)	16	Of which saturates (g)	0.5
Salt (g)	0.03	Fibre (g)	1.5

Serves 4
Prep time – 5–10 mins

1 nice ripe pineapple, chilled in the fridge
1 tbsp runny honey or maple syrup
bunch of fresh mint, chopped, plus a few whole leaves for decoration
squeeze of lemon juice
small handful toasted cashew nuts, roughly chopped

1. Prepare the pineapple – slice off the leafy plume and the stem, stand the pineapple upright on a cutting board and slice off the tough skin, following the curve of the fruit from top to bottom, then remove any extra bits left over, the 'eyes'.
2. Place the fruit on its side and then cut it into very thin slices with the sharpest knife you own.
3. Cut the slices in half and cut out the woody core.
4. Reserve the juice.
5. Lay the slices on 4 large flat plates.

6. Mix together the honey, the reserved pineapple juice, lemon juice and the mint and pour over the pineapple. Decorate with mint leaves and a few toasted nuts.
7. If you make this in advance, cut the pineapple and keep it in a bowl in the fridge, well covered with clingfilm, and then prepare from step 5 just before serving.

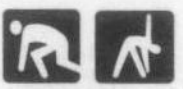

Recovery Rice Pudding

High G.I. Recovery 'Comfort' Food.

Short-grain 'pudding' rice has a very high G.I. and is a great way to get a serious amount of carbohydrate into your system after an event like a triathlon or marathon or after one of your big training sessions. There are hundreds of different recipes for rice pudding and everyone has their particular likes and dislikes – some adore the skin, some hate it; some like it cold, some hot. Whilst still fairly traditional, this recipe uses semi-skimmed milk and no butter, but don't worry, it is still really creamy. You can cook it the fast way to avoid skin or bake it slowly in the oven; you can even keep it in the fridge to attack as soon as you get home.

Nutrition per serving

Energy (kcal)	250	Protein (g)	10
Carbohydrate (g)	44	Fat (g)	5
Of which sugars (g)	23	Of which saturates (g)	3
Salt (g)	0.3	Fibre (g)	neg

Serves 4

Prep time – 2 minutes/Cooking time – 1½ hours

100g short-grain pudding rice
1 litre semi-skimmed milk
2 tbsp caster sugar
1 tsp demerara to serve
good grating of nutmeg
½–1 tsp cinnamon (or 1 cinnamon stick)
1 bay leaf (optional)

Method One – creamed rice

1. Mix all the ingredients together in a heavy-bottomed saucepan and bring to the boil.
2. Simmer on the lowest heat possible, using a diffuser if you have

one, for about 1–1¼ hours, until the rice has absorbed the milk and the texture is thick and creamy.

3. Sprinkle with a little demerara sugar to serve.

Method Two – rice pudding

1. Preheat the oven to 180°C/gas mark 4.
2. Mix all the ingredients in a lightly buttered oven dish and place in the oven.
3. After 30 minutes, stir to prevent the rice sticking together.
4. Turn the oven down to 150°C/gas mark 2, sprinkle a little sugar on the top and bake for another 1½ hours until a lovely brown skin has formed on the surface.

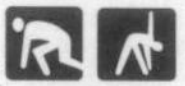

Stem Ginger and Poppy Seed Muffins

Great post-workout snack; these muffins will give you a boost.

One of my favourite stories to read the children when they were younger was *A Busy Day for a Good Grandmother*, a book from New Zealand about the perilous journey of Mrs Oberon, an intrepid grandmother who overcomes the Rif-Raf Rapids, braves alligators in the Swagwallow Swamp and fights off ice-vultures by shooting her healthy – but rather heavy – carrot muffins from the muffin ejector tube of her Piper Cherokee. Weighed down by the muffins, the ice-vultures lose altitude and Mrs Oberon manages to deliver her 'cock-a-hoop honey cake' to her teething grandson. Well, despite being healthy, I can guarantee that these muffins will not weigh you down. They are light and airy and very tasty. The secret is to make them quickly and to avoid over mixing – simply fold the wet ingredients into the dry until they are just combined and then pop them into the oven. Ginger is a great anti-inflammatory and can help reduce muscle spasms, while poppy seeds are a good source of important minerals such as thiamin, magnesium, phosphorous, zinc and copper – you'll find them in the supermarket alongside the packs of seeds, nuts and dried fruit.

Nutrition per serving

Energy (kcal)	329	Protein (g)	6
Carbohydrate (g)	47	Fat (g)	14
Of which sugars (g)	23	Of which saturates (g)	1.5
Salt (g)	0.5	Fibre (g)	2

Makes 12 big muffins
Prep time – 10 minutes/Cooking time – 30 minutes

200g white self-raising flour
200g wholemeal self-raising flour
pinch of salt
1 tsp ground ginger
1 tsp bicarbonate of soda

2 tsp baking powder
60g (3–4 lumps) preserved stem ginger, sliced finely and cut into thin strips
2 tbsp poppy seeds
75g soft brown sugar
75g golden caster sugar
2 eggs
150ml sunflower oil
1 tbsp stem ginger syrup or runny honey
1 ripe banana, peeled and mashed
125ml skimmed milk
125ml low-fat natural yoghurt
1 tbsp chopped stem ginger mixed with 1 tbsp demerera sugar to sprinkle on top

1. Preheat the oven to 180°C/gas mark 4 and line a muffin tray with 12 muffin cases.
2. Mix the two flours, salt, ground ginger, bicarbonate of soda and baking powder together.
3. Mix together the stem ginger and the poppy seeds and combine with the flour.
4. Put the sugar into a separate bowl, break in the eggs and then add the oil, syrup or honey, banana, milk and yoghurt.
5. Beat very lightly with a fork then pour the mixture into the bowl with the dry ingredients and combine quickly. The mixture will appear lumpy but don't worry, just spoon it into the muffin cases, sprinkle a little demerera sugar and ginger on top of each muffin and pop them into the oven for 30 minutes.
6. Remove from the oven, cool on a wire rack and eat immediately.

drinks and smoothies

'Always make sure you're well hydrated and remember it takes 72 hours or so to fully hydrate yourself, so start early.' Adam Bardsley, Managing Director, Ironman (personal best: 10:28) and marathon (personal best: 2:41) runner. Best event – Ironman France 2008.

'Synchronized swimming means you're in the pool and often upside down for long periods of time, so you can't have anything too heavy that'll sit in the bottom of your stomach. I also find that I'm performing early in the morning and it's hard for me to eat anything solid, and so I'll have lots of energy drinks.' Alex O'Mahony, synchronized swimmer, national champion in team and duet.

Avocado and Cucumber Lassi

Nutritionally balanced power drink, good for a boost before exercise or for rehydrating and replenishing lost nutrients after exercise. You could also make it for lunch in place of a solid meal.

A 'lassi' is an Indian yoghurt drink – the Indian version of a smoothie, really. It tends to be made with thick creamy yoghurt, but I find that the avocado makes it creamy enough, so I use a mix of low-fat yoghurt and skimmed milk. A fantastic way to drink your veggies, this is a high-energy power drink, yet the addition of the mint and the cucumber makes it taste light and fresh. Avocado is one of those superfoods which is just brimming with goodness – it has plenty of energy-giving calories, but they are the type of calories you want to put in your body. It is rich in potassium, B vitamins, beta-carotene and monounsaturated fats, which can help lower cholesterol and reduce blood pressure. What's more, the yoghurt/milk mix provides good amounts of calcium and protein. Depending on your mood and the time of day, you could give the drink a bit of kick with some spices such as ginger, coriander or cumin.

Nutrition per serving

Energy (kcal)	130	Protein (g)	5
Carbohydrate (g)	8	Fat (g)	8
Of which sugars (g)	7	Of which saturates (g)	2
Salt (g)	0.5	Fibre (g)	3

Makes 2 glasses
Prep time – 5 mins

½ avocado, chilled, peeled, stone removed and cut into cubes
½ cucumber, chilled, peeled and cut into cubes
pinch of salt
6 fresh mint leaves
75ml skimmed milk
75ml low-fat natural yoghurt

8 ice cubes
ground cumin and a stick of cucumber or fresh ginger to serve

1. Blend together the avocado, cucumber, salt, mint, milk and yoghurt in a blender.
2. Add the ice cubes and blend again until the ice is crushed.
3. Serve in tall glasses with some ground cumin sprinkled on top and a stick of cucumber or fresh ginger.

Banana, Mango and Pineapple Power Smoothie

A low- to medium-G.I. power drink, full of essential vitamins and minerals, which will keep you alert and full of energy for hours.

The marriage of mango, banana, pineapple and lime is one that really is made in heaven. Not only does it conjure up images of tropical beaches, but it also provides a hefty portion of beta-carotene, folic acid, fibre, vitamins B, C and E and essential minerals. The skimmed milk also adds protein and calcium. For peak health and vitality, this smoothie will give you that extra zest for life. If you can, chill all the ingredients first.

Nutrition per serving

Energy (kcal)	180	Protein (g)	4
Carbohydrate (g)	40	Fat (g)	1
Of which sugars (g)	40	Of which saturates (g)	Neg
Salt (g)	0.1	Fibre (g)	4.5

Makes 2 glasses
Prep time – 5 minutes

8 ice cubes
1 ripe mango, peeled, stoned and chopped
½ fresh pineapple, peeled, cored and chopped
1 small banana or ½ a large banana, chopped
Juice of ½–1 lime (according to taste)
150ml skimmed milk

1. Crush the ice cubes in the blender and then add the rest of the ingredients.
2. Blend until smooth.
3. If the smoothie is too thick, add a little more cold milk.

Beetroot, Apple, Carrot and Watercress Iron Boost

Delicious and fresh tasting, this juice will give you a real boost if you are feeling low or under the weather, and it is brimming with vitamins, iron and disease-fighting nutrients.

This juice is packed with iron, folic acid, essential minerals and antioxidants. What is more, the vitamin C in the vegetables and the apple juice helps your body to absorb the iron. The watercress adds a lovely spicy, peppery taste and balances the sweetness of the carrot and beetroot. You might find the purple colour of the juice a little unusual, but latest research suggests that purple foods such as beetroot can protect you against heart disease, strokes, cancer and Alzheimer's disease. Give it a go, you'll be pleasantly surprised.

Nutrition per serving

Energy (kcal)	62	Protein (g)	1.5
Carbohydrate (g)	14	Fat (g)	0.5
Of which sugars (g)	13	Of which saturates (g)	Neg
Salt (g)	0.1	Fibre (g)	2

Makes 2 glasses
Prep time – 5 minutes

1 small cooked beetroot (about 50g)
1 large carrot, peeled
150ml apple juice
100ml water
4–5 ice cubes
handful of watercress (remove any thick stalks)
pinch of salt and freshly ground black pepper

1. Chop the carrot and the beetroot into small cubes and put in a blender with the apple juice, water and the ice cubes.
2. Blend for a minute. Add the watercress and blend again until the mixture is really smooth.
3. Add a pinch of salt and some black pepper. Strain the juice through a tea strainer or sieve.

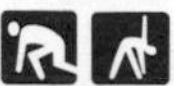

Ginger and Melon Rescue Remedy

Rehydrating and refreshing recovery drink for after exercise.

Melon has a higher G.I. than most fruit; it has a high water content and it is particularly refreshing. Athletes will often eat melon to recover and rehydrate straight after a long workout. Ginger is known for its anti-inflammatory qualities, so make up this juice in advance and enjoy it as soon as you get back from your hot and sweaty 17-mile training run.

Nutrition per serving

Energy (kcal)	50	Protein (g)	1.5
Carbohydrate (g)	10	Fat (g)	Neg
Of which sugars (g)	10	Of which saturates (g)	Neg
Salt (g)	0.05	Fibre (g)	2.5

Makes 2 glasses
Prep time – 5 minutes

1 chilled melon (gala, charentais, honeydew – it works well with any type except watermelon), skinned and deseeded
small piece of fresh ginger (½–1cm), peeled and chopped
4 ice cubes
sprig of mint and a long piece of ginger to serve

1. Scoop out the flesh from the melon.
2. Put the melon, ginger and the ice cubes into a blender and whiz until smooth
3. Serve in a tall glass with a sprig of mint and a long piece of ginger as a stirrer.

Pear and Watercress Wake-up Juice

A low-G.I. refreshing breakfast drink, full of essential vitamins and minerals to keep you alert and full of energy for hours.

This juice is perfect to wake you up first thing in the morning and goes down very well with a date and walnut breakfast muffin (see page 64). Rich in vitamins C, B1, B6, K and E, beta-carotene, anti-oxidants and essential minerals such as zinc, magnesium, manganese, calcium and potassium, this juice really is a 'super-drink'. The pear adds sweetness to the peppery watercress, and also helps your body absorb the iron. It has long been known that water-cress is good for you. Apparently, the Greek general Xenophon gave his soldiers watercress to increase their vigour before going into battle and the Egyptian pharaohs gave their slaves freshly squeezed watercress juice to increase their productivity.

Nutrition per serving

Energy (kcal)	90	Protein (g)	1
Carbohydrate (g)	22	Fat (g)	0.5
Of which sugars (g)	22	Of which saturates (g)	Neg
Salt (g)	0.03	Fibre (g)	3

Makes 2 glasses
Prep time – 5 minutes

2 ripe chilled pears, peeled, cored and chopped
large handful of watercress, thick stalks removed
200ml apple juice
4 ice cubes
¼ tsp ground ginger (optional)

1. Whiz everything together in a blender until smooth.
2. Pour through a strainer into two long glasses and drink immediately.

Strawberry Mint Vitamin Rush

Vitamin-rich energy drink to give you a boost at any time of day, before exercise or for rehydration after exercise, or if you just want to indulge yourself.

Just the colour of this vivid red juice should wake you up and put a smile on your face. Rich in beta-carotene, folic acid, biotin, vitamin C, minerals and small amounts of B vitamins, this juice not only tastes fantastic, but will also make you feel alert and ready to take on the world.

Nutrition per serving

Energy (kcal)	82	Protein (g)	1
Carbohydrate (g)	20	Fat (g)	0.5
Of which sugars (g)	19	Of which saturates (g)	Neg
Salt (g)	0.02	Fibre (g)	1.5

Makes 2 glasses
Prep time – 5 minutes

20–30 strawberries (about 200–250g), stalks removed
200ml apple juice
½ tsp balsamic vinegar
½ tsp icing sugar
½ kiwi fruit (optional)
4 ice cubes
4 mint leaves, plus a sprig to decorate

1. Put everything into the blender and whiz until smooth.
2. Pour into two long glasses and decorate with a couple of mint leaves.

Tomato Chilli Zinger

Nutritious savoury drink, great for replacing lost salts after exercise or if you need to give yourself a quick booster. Also makes a tasty, non-alcoholic cocktail.

This drink is absolutely packed with vitamins and minerals and the little added spice is perfect if you need to give yourself a kick-start. If you are feeling low or lethargic, or if you have just come back from a big training session, try a glass of this.

Nutrition per serving

Energy (kcal)	40	Protein (g)	2
Carbohydrate (g)	7.5	Fat (g)	1
Of which sugars (g)	7	Of which saturates (g)	Neg
Salt (g)	1	Fibre (g)	2

Makes 2 glasses
Prep time – 5 minutes

250ml tomato juice
½ red pepper, deseeded
¼ small red chilli, deseeded and chopped
5cm piece of cucumber, peeled
½ stick of celery, stringy bits removed
salt and freshly ground black pepper
squeeze of lemon
dash of Tabasco and Worcestershire sauce to taste
4 ice cubes
basil leaves and celery stick to decorate

1. Blend everything together in a blender. Taste for seasoning.
2. Serve in tall glasses with some basil leaves and a celery stick as a stirrer.

menu plan suggestions

These menu plans are designed to suit most endurance sports, whether you are a long distance runner or cyclist, a triathlete, a rower or a swimmer. They include three meals a day, plus snacks, and aim to give an example of how you can use the recipes provided in the book to keep your glycogen and energy levels on an even keel, thus minimising the urge to stoke up on processed foods, munch through endless packets of biscuits and raid the office vending machine for chocolate bars and crisps.

3-day example menu plan for general endurance training

Go Faster tips

- *Base your meals on those with a low glycaemic index to promote efficient glycogen refuelling and more sustained energy levels.*
- *Eat healthy snacks between meals to prevent dips in energy.*
- *Eat or drink a high-G.I. snack or meal immediately after exercise.*
- *Drink regularly.*
- *Eat well on recovery days.*

Day one

Breakfast
Spiced autumn fruits with crunchy granola and low-fat natural yoghurt
Slice of wholemeal toast with your favourite spread
Glass of fruit juice
Snack
Lunch
Hummus and rocket sandwich
Slice of carrot cake
Snack
Supper
Conchiglioni with roasted tomato sauce
Green salad

Day two

Breakfast
Banana, mango and pineapple smoothie
Slice of wholemeal toast with your favourite spread
Snack
Lunch
Lemon basil spaghetti
Piece of fruit
Snack
Supper
Roasted butternut squash risotto
Green bean salad

Day three

Breakfast
Go Faster porridge with walnuts and blueberries
Glass of orange juice
Snack
Lunch
Butter bean soup with crispy pancetta
Crusty granary roll
Snack
Supper
Thai green fish curry with rice noodles

Big endurance Sunday – meal plan for your weekend endurance session of 90 minutes or more

Go Faster tips

- *If you are planning an early morning endurance session, like a 16 mile run or a long cycle ride, get up 1–1½ hours before you plan to set off, drink a pint of water and eat breakfast immediately.*
- *Eat a post-workout recovery snack as soon as you get back.*

Saturday night meal

Couscous with chicken tagine, preserved lemon and green olives
Almond tarta di Santiago
Or
Lemon and fennel pilaf with garlic prawns
Fruit salad and low-fat yoghurt with granola sprinkles

Sunday

Pre-workout breakfast

Go faster porridge with honey, nuts and raisins

Mid-morning post-workout recovery

Ginger and melon rescue remedy
American blueberry pancake

Lunch

Roasted parsnip soup with cumin and chilli
Stem ginger and poppyseed muffin
Or
Recovery rice pudding

Supper

Pink peppercorn risotto with pork and peanuts
Green salad
Pineapple carpaccio with mint
Or
Red curry duck with lychees and fragrant jasmine rice
Poached nectarines and vanilla ricotta cream

Gearing up to an event – for high-intensity events of over 90 minutes

Go Faster tips

- *Aim to eat 8–10g carbohydrate per kg of body weight per day, especially in the three days leading up to the event.*
- *Eat three good meals a day, plus a morning and afternoon snack.*
- *Drink copiously during the week before the event, so that your body is really well hydrated. Aim for three litres per day.*
- *You may start to feel less hungry, as you will have tapered your training – try to keep up the carbohydrate and eat less protein and fat.*
- *Stick to plain, familiar food the day before the event and don't overeat.*

Day one

Breakfast
Bowl of Weetabix
Banana
Glass of orange juice
1–2 slices of wholemeal toast with your favourite spread
Lunch
Chickpea falafel or Lebanese couscous salad
Supper
Pappardelle with scallops, broad beans, bacon and mint

Day two

Breakfast
Devilled tomatoes on toast
Pear and water-cress wake-up juice
Lunch
Lemon basil spaghetti
Supper
Smoky black bean and chorizo chilli salsa

Day three

Breakfast
Scrambled eggs with either wholemeal toast or drop scones
Glass of fruit juice
Lunch
Butter bean soup with crispy pancetta
Supper
Algerian chicken and apricot tagine with plain couscous

Day four

Breakfast
Birchermuesli or porridge with fruit
1–2 slices of wholemeal toast with your favourite spread
Glass of orange juice
Lunch
Butternut squash risotto
Supper
Chickpea, sweet potato and spinach soup
Crusty wholemeal bread
Frisée salad with oven roasted walnuts

Day five

Breakfast
Fruit and nut muesli with banana and low fat yoghurt
1–2 slices of wholemeal toast with your favourite spread
Glass of juice
Lunch
Farfalle pasta with roasted artichokes
Supper
Spicy chicken and chickpea pilaf with yoghurt and cucumber sauce, chutney and naan bread
Fresh baby leaf spinach salad

Day six

Breakfast
Breton buckwheat pancakes with ham and cheese
Glass of orange juice
Lunch
Fillet of salmon with green couscous
Supper
Spaghetti with toasted pine nuts, fresh basil and parmesan
Tomato salad

Day seven – competition day

Remember, DON'T consume anything you are not used to

Breakfast – about 3 hours before race start
Go Faster Porridge with blueberries, honey and walnuts
Slice of wholemeal toast with your favourite jam, honey or peanut butter
Pint of water or a light smoothie like a strawberry mint vitamin rush

Lunch (if event is not until the afternoon)
Conchiglioni with tomato sauce
Glass of apple juice
500ml water

1–1½ hours before race
Bottle of sports drink
Banana, flapjack or a honey or peanut butter sandwich on wholemeal bread

Recommended snacks for during race (for instance, if you are cycling, between heats or on endurance fell run)
Fresh fruit e.g. banana or an orange cut into slices
Malty fruit loaf or flapjack
Handful of dried fruit and/or nuts and seeds
Sports drink
Jelly babies/sports beans/glucose tablets
Energy gels
Marmite sandwich

Post-event snack
Bottle of water or sports drink
Piece of higher G.I. fruit such as melon or a bottle of smoothie
Chocolate biscuit cake
Walnut and white chocolate chip brownie

Post-event meal
Penang prawn curry with fragrant steamed jasmine rice
Date tart with cardamom and orange flower water
Or
Gnocchi with mushroom sauce, rocket and parmesan salad
Recovery rice pudding
Or
Creamy risotto of broad beans, mint and pancetta
Chocolate pecan tart

Lunches 'on the run'

It's not so easy to just throw together a bowl of pasta when you are away from home or out all day at work. A healthy sandwich followed by a piece of fruit and a flapjack makes a perfect training lunch when you are out and about.

Go Faster tips

- *Don't skip meals. Try to think ahead, take your own healthy sandwiches or pasta salads to work with you or choose ready-made lunches carefully.*
- *Use good bread, rolls or pitta – wholemeal, granary, seeded brown, olive bread, wholemeal pitta or wraps.*
- *Use only a small amount of butter or mayonnaise, or leave it out completely.*
- *If you are buying lunch, go to a sandwich shop and have the sandwich made in front of you. Avoid high-fat fillings like coronation chicken and prawn mayo.*
- *Baked potatoes are a great 'on-the-go' alternative to sandwiches.*

Try these healthy sandwich fillings:

- Smoked salmon, low-fat cream cheese and rocket with black pepper
- Chicken and pesto
- Chicken, lettuce and tomato
- Chargrilled chicken and sunblush tomatoes
- Hummus and rocket
- Tuna or prawns, watercress, plenty of black pepper and a light spreading of mayonnaise
- Low-fat soft cheese, parma ham, dates and walnuts
- Low-fat soft cheese with grated celery, raisins and carrot
- Avocado, grated carrot and watercress with plenty of salt and pepper
- Little gem lettuce, finely sliced cheddar cheese, mango chutney

- Pastrami, gherkin and wholegrain mustard
- Left-over roast beef, rocket and horseradish

Healthy Snacks

Burning so many calories during a training schedule, it is important to eat at regular intervals throughout the day and especially before and after your workouts. This will maintain steady blood sugar and glycogen levels.

Pre-workout snacks

- Nuts, raisins, dates, dried apricots and seeds
- Fruit cake
- Energy oat or granola bars and malt loaf
- 'Healthy' wholemeal muffins
- Fruit or fruit salad
- Banana sandwich on wholemeal bread
- Peanut butter sandwich (wholemeal bread)
- Hummus and pitta bread

From *Go Faster Food* recipes

- Strawberry mint vitamin rush
- Banana, mango and pineapple smoothie
- Avocado and cucumber lassi
- Date and walnut muffin
- Handful of granola
- Date, apricot and walnut flapjacks
- Mincemeat and orange flapjacks
- Honey, ginger and lime oaties
- Go Faster carrot cake
- Malty fruit bars

Post-workout snacks

- Honey sandwich (white bread)
- Rice cakes with honey, jam or marmite

- Cantaloupe melon
- Banana cake
- Energy bars and malt loaf
- Low-fat yoghurt and honey
- A few pieces of dark chocolate
- Handful of chocolate raisins

From *Go Faster Food* recipes

- Ginger and melon rescue remedy
- Tomato and chilli zinger
- Chocolate panforte
- Chocolate biscuit cake
- Orange marmalade cake
- Stem ginger and poppyseed muffins
- Walnut and white chocolate brownies
- Recovery rice pudding
- Handful of granola
- Date, apricot and walnut flapjacks
- Mincemeat and orange flapjacks
- Honey, ginger and lime oaties

store cupboard suggestions

I have had several requests on my gofasterfood blog (http://gofasterfood.blogspot.com) for a list of foods I would normally keep in my cupboard. One blogger complains that he has spent the past 20 years coming back from the shops with bags of stuff which either end up in the bin or tucked away at the back of the shelf. Well, I can guarantee that he is not the only one – there are all sorts of unusual specialities at the back of my cupboards: pickled aubergines, piri piri powder, a vacuum pack of dried shrimp to name but a few. However, keeping a healthy stash of both interesting and standard foods in your store cupboard, fridge and freezer and buying some staple, longer lasting vegetables not only means there is always a standby meal to be made, but it also makes for a fun and varied diet. You will find that you will develop your own 'interesting' store cupboard as you increase your range of recipes. Remember to keep your fruit bowl well stocked as well and buy fresh ingredients whenever possible.

Here is my list of some useful Go Faster store cupboard essentials:

Dried food essentials

- **Pasta** – keep a variety of different types, wholemeal and white spaghetti, conchiglioni, twirls, bows, bucatini etc.
- **Rice** – basmati, brown basmati, arborio, vialone nano, red rice, wild rice, pudding rice, Thai fragrant jasmine rice

- **Grains** – couscous, polenta, bulgur wheat, pearl barely, Riso Gallo 3-grain, quinoa
- **Lentils and pulses** – bags of beans for overnight soaking, such as butter beans, haricot, flageolet, chickpeas, black beans
- **Noodles** – Thai rice noodles, soba noodles, egg noodles
- **Whole rolled unrefined porridge oats** – these are the best for endurance
- **Dried fruit and nuts** – keep bags of different varieties: dates, apricots, raisins, figs, flaked almonds, whole almonds, Brazil nuts, walnuts, pecans and cashews, pine nuts, sunflower seeds, pumpkin seeds
- **Dark chocolate** – this always makes its way to the front of my cupboard
- **Rice cakes, oatcakes**
- **Flour** – self-raising and plain, wholemeal and white, buckwheat

Jars and tins

- **Tomatoes** – chopped tomatoes, passata, sugocasa, tomato puree
- **Baked beans** – sometimes baked beans on toast really hits the spot
- **Lentils and pulses** – kidney beans, chickpeas to make a quick hummus, flageolet beans, butter beans, red lentils for speedy soups
- **Oily fish** – tuna, sardines, anchovies
- **Interesting oils** – cold-pressed extra-virgin olive, light olive for cooking, rapeseed, walnut, pumpkin seed, sunflower
- **Vinegars** – balsamic, white balsamic, white and red wine, cider
- **Sugar replacements** – manuka honey, maple syrup, molasses, golden syrup, malt extract
- **Jars of curry paste** – madras, penang, Thai green and red curry paste
- **Chutneys, minced chillies, minced ginger, tamarind**
- **Coconut milk and coconut cream**
- **Tasty jars of antipasti** – olives, sunblush/sun-dried tomatoes, roasted artichokes

- **Interesting preserved foods in brine** – preserved lemons, capers, pink/green peppercorns
- **Mustards** – whole grain, Dijon, English

Freezer

- **Vegetables** – peas, spinach, broad beans
- **Fish** – tiger prawns, scallops, shrimps, salmon steaks
- **Fresh pasta** – lasagne, tagliatelle
- **Fresh gnocchi**
- **Fruit** – summer fruits, blueberries, fruit for smoothies
- **Pitta bread, wholemeal rolls**
- **Essentials for Thai food are great kept in the freezer** – kaffir lime leaves, lemon grass, ginger

Herbs, spices and specials

- **Dried herbs** – mixed herbs, thyme, oregano, rosemary, basil, tarragon, sage
- **Spices** – coriander, cumin, fennel, garam masala, cardamom, star anise, ras-el-hanout, Moroccan spice, ginger, cinnamon sticks, mixed spice, ground cinnamon, juniper berries, cloves, saffron, paprika, chilli powder, Spanish smoked paprika
- **Specials** – orange flower water, rose water

Vegetable Rack

- **Garlic**
- **Ginger**
- **Longer lasting vegetables** – butternut squash, potatoes, parsnips, pumpkin, carrots, onions, fennel, celery, peppers, savoy cabbage, red cabbage, beetroot (buy other veg and fresh herbs as and when you need them)

index